Why Does My Back Hurt So Much?

A comprehensive guide to help you prevent and treat lower back pain

Why Does My Back Hurt So Much?

A comprehensive guide to help you prevent and treat lower back pain

Mark Amir MAPT, Dip. MDT
Perry Bonomo MAPT

ErgAerobics, Inc. New York

Written By:

Mark Amir MAPT, Dip. MDT & Perry Bonomo MAPT

Manufactured: USA

ISBN: 0966409019

Library of Congress Card Number: 00-110948

Editing: Paul Winter, Tamar Friedman, Steven Kletzkin

Medical Illustrations: Paul Winter

Graphic Design: Austin Bass, Alyssa Law

Photographs: Dean Hansen

Book Design: Shawn Andringa

Cover Design: Brian Pieters/Masterfile

Model: Joy DeJager

Madison Spine & Physical Therapy

3311 Shore Parkway, Suite FF

Brooklyn, NY 11235

Tel: 888.457.4575

E-mail: perryergaerobics@yahoo.com

Web site: www.ergaerobics.com

DEDICATION

This book is dedicated to the following important people in our lives:

My parents, who are my role models and heroes. My brothers, Boaz, Avner and Eytan, who challenge me to exceed perfection. My new and extended family Vera and Ari, who believe in me and encourage me to fulfill my dreams. My father -in-law Sasha, your wisdom is irreplaceable. My sons, Alexander and Jonathan, my newest bundles of joy. Most important, to my wife and best friend, you have made my life heaven without borders.

-Mark

My wife, who is the backbone of my spirit and desire to do well. My son Casey, I love you more than I could ever imagine. My parents, whose unconditional love and support enable me to succeed. My brother, Steve, and his wife, Dianc, who always believe in me and to all of my in-laws, thank you for your support and encouragement.

To my Grandma Ruth, I miss you. You were the greatest.

-Perry

Table of Contents

FOREWORD

The most common complaint of patients in our clinic is back pain. In fact, according to national statistics, 4 out of 5 people in this country will experience severe lower back pain at some time in their lives. We have spent much time wondering why so many people suffer from back pain. Is back pain preventable? Can people treat themselves for back pain and avoid expensive medical treatments? The answers are in this book. After years of research, we have concluded that pain medications, modalities and frequent manipulations are not the answers. Nothing will keep you as healthy and pain-free as what you can easily do in the comfort of your own home or at work. The way you work, sit, stand, lift and drive are just a few of the behaviors that could lead to back pain. By being more aware of these behaviors, you will likely avoid an episode of severe back pain. If these same activities are done improperly, the likelihood for you to become a part of the population with back pain is dramatically increased.

We decided to write this book to help you take care of your back. We realize that the majority of people do not know how to properly take care of their back. People generally perform harmful movements until the day comes when they injure their back. At that point, they usually seek outside care. They may go to their doctor to receive pain medication or to their chiropractor for manipulations. Commonly, they will feel better in a couple of days and then go back to their daily routine. Unfortunately, many people fall into a cycle of pain if they don't change their daily routine. They usually end up injuring their back again! But this time, their back injury takes a little longer to heal. This cycle will repeat itself over and over again. Sometimes it will take several years for the cycle to repeat. More often the second and third injuries happen within months or even weeks of each other. The vicious cycle of pain has begun. The patient becomes dependent on the medical community for his or her well being and is left with little to no control.

The goal of this book is to teach you how to take care of your back so that you no longer need to rely solely on the medical community to make you feel better. We will teach you how to modify your behavior to place less strain on your back during your daily activities. You will soon understand why poor postural behaviors can cause back pain and how to avoid these behaviors. Exercise for your back will no longer become a chore but a part of your everyday activity. You do not need expensive equipment or a gym to help you stay healthy! Our exercises will become part of your daily routine. After reading this book, you will become knowledgeable on how to treat your back.

To keep the material light and interesting, we created a few animated characters: Sergio, who represents safety and ergonomics; Muskull, who represents muscle pain; Disco, who represents disc problems; and Nervie, who represents nerve pain. You will read about the trials and tribulations they suffer after they injure themselves, and then how, with Sergio's help, they took care of their backs. Their stories might remind you of some of the problems you have encountered.

Our goal is to have a healthier and happier you. We hope you enjoy this book and take away with you a few helpful hints on how to prevent and treat lower back pain.

Mark and Perry

INTRODUCTION

Will it make you feel any better to know that if your back hurts you are not alone? Eighty percent of the population at one time or another has experienced back pain. Each year businesses spend $100 billion treating lower back pain. Back pain treatment is at epidemic proportions. What can be done to stop this epidemic?

We can help you avoid lower back pain. There are ways to detect early warning signs of back pain. These warning signs can help you identify a small problem and prevent it from becoming a big one. We will teach you what these warning signs are and how to minimize the frequency and progression of a back injury.

Unlike a broken arm or leg, back injuries often stem from a repetitious cycle of seemingly harmless everyday movements. It is necessary to look at how you perform your everyday normal activities. Do you slouch when you sit or stand? Do you bend your knees when you lift things from the floor? How do you sit while driving, eating, or even relaxing?

Generally, people wait until they sustain an injury to change their behaviors. It is difficult to convince people that constant slouching will cause them back pain. It is difficult to change the way people lift if they have never experienced the constant, often disabling pain that comes with a back injury.

We've found that many of our patients have presented with similar complaints of back pain. After researching our treatments for these patients, we came to an important conclusion: **Most of the problems we treat are preventable.** Through proper education about body mechanics, you can take steps both at work and at home, to dramatically decrease your risk of a debilitating back injury. We decided to put our oral advice in print. Our goal is to have a back pain-free society. We will tell you how incorporating simple exercises to your daily routine can help minimize the chances of developing disabling back pain.

The prevention of back pain can be compared to the maintenance of an automobile. If you neglect to maintain the automobile by changing the oil, replacing the tires and brakes or tuning the engine, the automobile will stop operating efficiently. The same is true of the human body. If you neglect to maintain it by exercising, eating nutritiously and resting, it will stop operating efficiently.

The majority of you who read this book will have already suffered a back injury and are looking for the answers. This book will teach you how to take care of yourself by modifying your behavior. We will teach you the proper way to perform your daily activities in order to preserve the life of your back. What at first might have felt awkward to you will now become second nature to you. Soon the roles of good behavior and bad behavior will be reversed. Bad behavioral habits will now feel awkward and good behavioral habits will feel normal. The change of your behavior will result in a healthier, pain-free you.

Chapter 1

Why Does My Back Hurt So Much?

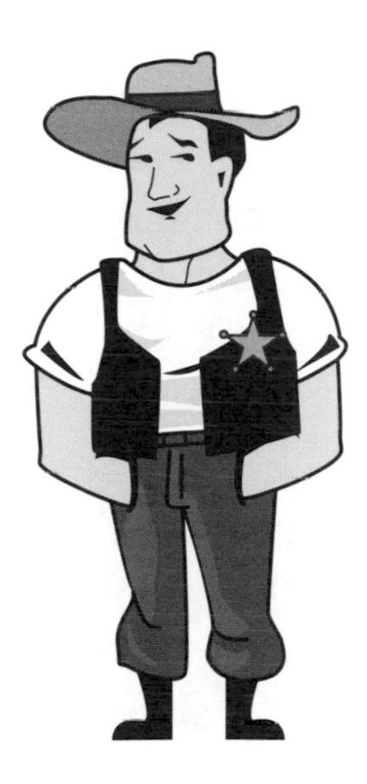

Sergio (**S**afety & **ERG**onom**I**c **O**fficer) is an average guy working hard to achieve his American dream. A dream consisting of a wonderful wife and children, a job he enjoys and a paycheck that allows him and his family to live comfortably. After graduating college, Sergio married the love of his life and got a job as a computer programmer. A few years later, he and his wife started a family. Sergio began working longer hours to support his family. As expenses racked up, Sergio found himself working harder and harder, leaving little time for exercise and proper nutrition. By his mid-thirties he started to slow down. The years of sitting slouched in front of the computer, and lack of exercise and nutrition were taking their toll. One day, while working on an important assignment, Sergio experienced severe lower back pain. Realizing this would affect his job performance, he rushed to a doctor for treatment.

The doctor gave him pain medication. Sergio took the medication and in a couple of days he felt better. Sergio went back to his normal routine, happy that the pain was gone. A few weeks later, Sergio once again felt severe lower back pain. Sergio did not want to rely on pain medication for the rest of his life so this time he went to a chiropractor. Sergio left the chiropractor's office after he received lower back manipulations and went back to his normal routine. He felt much better. A few more weeks went by, and Sergio once again felt severe lower back pain. Rather than go to the doctor or the chiropractor Sergio decided to go see a physical therapist. The physical therapist performed electrical stimulation and ultrasound to his back. He walked out of the physical therapist's office feeling better and went back to his normal routine. A few weeks later, he experienced severe lower back pain again. Sergio had fallen into a vicious cycle of pain that he desperately wanted to get out of.

Sergio searched for the answers as to why he was in so much pain. He felt that he worked and lived like everyone else. What Sergio did not know was that the majority of the population has back pain. Sergio's curiosity drove him to watch people. He watched the habits of others and noticed that people performed their jobs differently. He noticed that some people, worked with good posture, used good body mechanics while lifting, ate right and exercised regularly, while others did not seem to care how they treated their body. Things started to make sense to Sergio. He noticed the difference in the people who took care of their body and those who did not. Those who took care of themselves seemed happier. They smiled most of the time and never complained of pain. What was their secret?

Then a friend of his told him that in order to feel better, he would have to change the way he did his normal activities. He gave Sergio a book entitled, Why Does My Back Hurt So Much? Curious, Sergio began to read this book. He slowly began to take steps to change his daily habits. He started incorporating the principles from the book into his daily routine and he immediately started feeling better. He was becoming one of the lucky people he observed. He was happier and more productive at work. He was patient with people, and everyone commented on how much healthier he looked.

Sergio felt great. With his renewed confidence he decided that it was time to change careers. Sergio opened a computer store. He was determined to create a healthy and productive environment for his workers. He preached the importance of working safely and encouraged exercising on the job. He demonstrated good body mechanics during lifting, and explained the importance of having good posture while sitting or standing. He set up his store ergonomically correct to minimize injuries on the job and to maintain a happier, healthier workplace.

Despite Sergio's efforts to have a healthy workplace, his employees were too stubborn to listen.

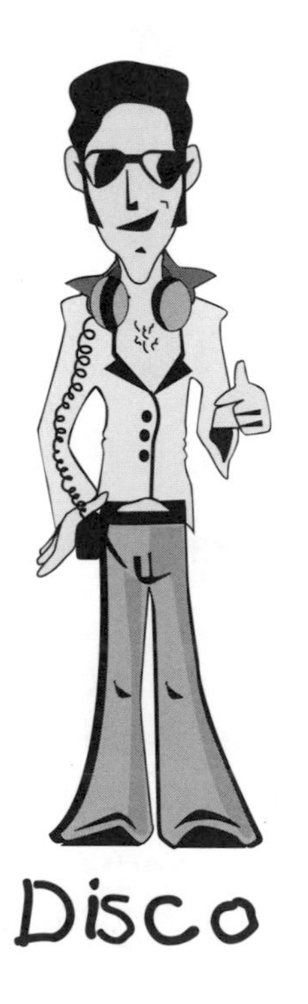

One of Sergio's charismatic employees was Disco. Disco was a throwback to the 70's. He would always dress in outrageous plaid and polyester outfits. He would blast his eight tracks of 70's dance music at work, much to the disgust of his co-workers, and would dance his way through the workday.

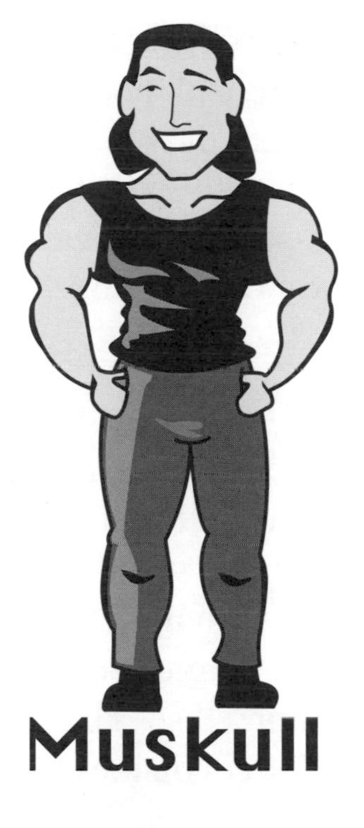

Muskull was another employee. Muskull was as vain as Disco was silly. Muskull, a weightlifting fanatic, was as strong as an ox and always enjoyed working in front of a mirror so that he could admire himself.

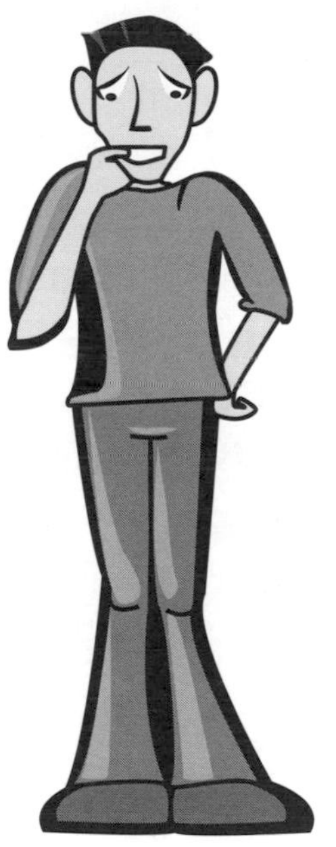

Nervie

Nervie, another employee, was nothing like Disco or Muskull. Nervie could never stand still and spoke a mile a minute. He would frequently interrupt Disco and Muskull to repeat a story he had already told.

Despite their shortcomings, Sergio was pleased with his staff. All three were young and felt invincible. Unfortunately, despite Sergio's warnings, they had no interest in taking care of their backs. After all, why fix something that is not broken.

Sergio was still concerned about his workers. He knew from reading Why Does My Back Hurt So Much? that chances were that if they continued to work with poor body mechanics and posture they would hurt their backs. Muskull and Disco did most of the lifting and manual labor. They moved inventory, set up workstations, and spent the majority of the day doing heavy work. Nervie's job was quite the opposite. Nervie sat in front of the computer and recorded inventory. The three men worked well together and Sergio was pleased with the success of his store.

But as fate would have it, in a span of three months, all three men began feeling back pain. Unfortunately, this occurred during the busiest time of year. Muskull was the first to get hurt: While loading boxes he pulled a muscle in his back. The workload then fell on Disco's hands. The long hours and heavy work slowed Disco up. The dancing and singing stopped and it was obvious that Disco was hurt. Sergio sent him home and told him to see a doctor. Disco was diagnosed with a bulging disc. The pressure at the store was great, and poor Nervie couldn't hang on. After countless hours in front of the computer, Nervie irritated his last good nerve.

Sergio was concerned for his employees and for his business. He had only three people working for him, and all of them were injured. Productivity was down and his business started to suffer. If that wasn't bad enough, his Workers Compensation insurance was on the rise and his profits no longer existed. What was once an up-and-coming business was now struggling to survive. Sergio was confused. Despite his efforts to set up the work environment ergonomically correct, Muskull, Nervie and Disco still suffered lower back pain. Knowing that the store was struggling, the three men tried their best to be productive. But Sergio was growing more frustrated each day. He finally decided to give them a book he now sold in his store entitled, Why Does My Back Hurt So Much? He instructed the three of them to read the book. Sergio believed the information was important for them to follow. He decided to take matters into his own hands and teach them the principles taught in this book. After all, it worked for him. Each day he provided them with helpful tips and healthy advice to help them through the workday. Sergio was so impressed with how simple it was to take care of his own back that he became an "expert" on preventing back injuries.

Chapter 2

General Exercise Rules for a Pain-free Back

Ever since Sergio discovered how a few simple exercises could help a person feel better, he has been trying to get everyone he knows to do them. His first hope was to get his workers Disco, Muskull and Nervie on an exercise program. He put up a sign that said **EXERCISE, EXERCISE AND MORE EXERCISE** at their workstations so that they could see it throughout the day. He incorporated three 15-minute exercise breaks, one in the morning, one at lunchtime and one at the end of the day into their work schedule. Nervie and Disco attended the exercise breaks but Muskull refused to. He thought he already knew every thing about exercise, since he lifted weights.

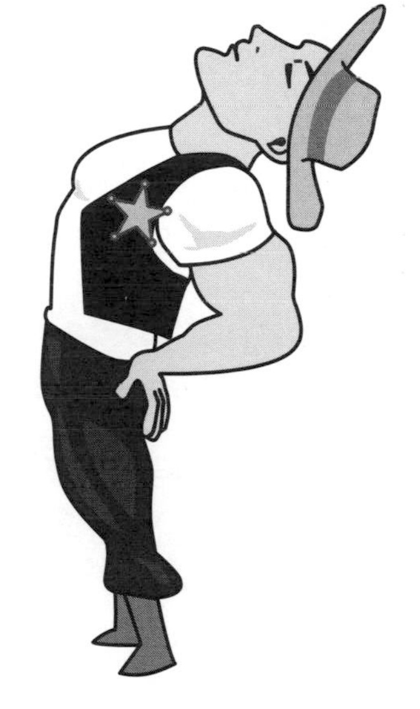

Muskull didn't know that there are 3 important types of exercises.

1. Stretching
2. Cardiovascular
3. Strengthening

Sergio: It is important to warm up your muscles before stretching. Fast walking indoors or outside, light jogging, biking, rowing, jumping jacks, jumping rope, or anything else that will make you breathe a little faster will warm up your muscles. (These are called **cardiovascular exercises.**) A good warm up will help you prevent injury when performing strengthening exercises. These are exercises that require the muscles to use a lot of their energy to move a weight. This can be in the form of a push up, sit up, squat etc.

Sergio's first order of business was to emphasize the importance of stretching properly.

Sergio: A stretch is an activity that holds a muscle in a position for a prolonged period of time, but before we stretch, it is important to follow these simple rules.

1. Start each stretch gradually. Stretch until you feel a slight discomfort and then relax.
2. Always stretch within your own limits. Do not compare yourself to others and try to stretch more.
3. Hold each stretch between 20 and 45 seconds.

4. It is important to stretch after a warm up and after completion of a sport or exercise regimen.
5. Breathe slowly and deeply when stretching. This should help you relax and give you a better stretch.

Nervie and Disco wanted to follow Sergio's stretching advice, however, they did not understand the importance of stretching. How could stretching cure their injuries? Finally, Nervie mustered up the nerve to ask Sergio.

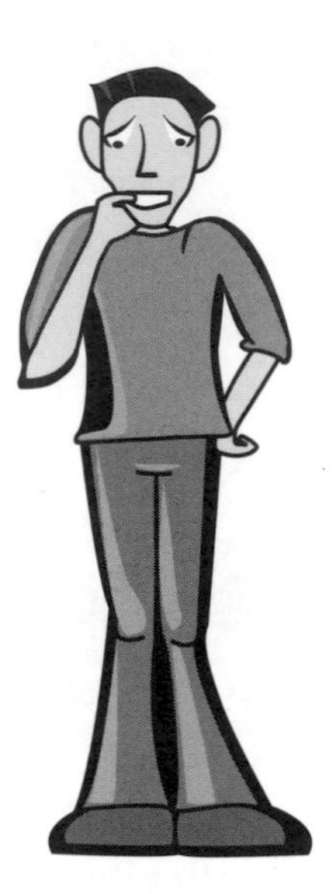

Nervie: WHY MUST WE STRETCH?

Sergio: Excellent question Nervie. These are the benefits your body will feel from stretching every day!

Stretching helps prevent muscle soreness from exercise or work activities. Stretching in the morning helps loosen up tight muscles and it allows your body to relax. Stretching reduces the likelihood of injuries and helps send blood and nutrients to the muscles. Stretching helps your body move without pain.

Now that Nervie and Disco understood the benefits of stretching and enjoyed their exercises, they both wanted to know more.

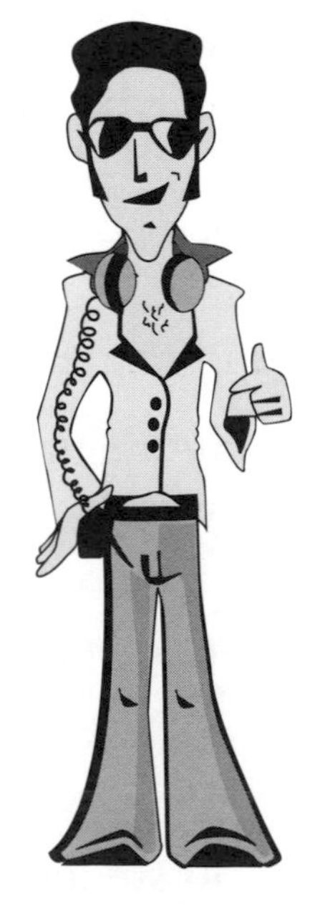

Disco: Is there anything we can do to strengthen our muscles?

Happy that Nervie and Disco were willing to change their behavior, Sergio told them how to strengthen their muscles.

Sergio: Sure Disco, there are several activities that you can do to strengthen your muscles. Strengthening is any activity that puts tension on the muscle to increase its ability to work. But first, there are some basic rules you need to follow.

1. Warm up first. Do five minutes of any of the following:

   Fast walking in place or outside, light jogging, biking, rowing, jumping jacks, jumping rope, or anything else that will make your heart beat a little faster.

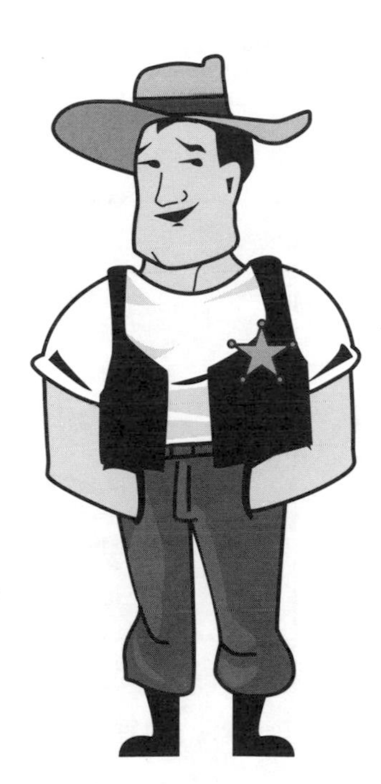

Sergio's Tip: "The Talk Test". You must be able to talk (or sing) during exercise! If not, your heart rate is probably too high.

2. Stretch whatever parts of your body you are about to strengthen.
3. All strengthening exercises should be done with good control. Do not jerk your body in any way during any strengthening exercise. Concern yourself more with the proper form than the amount of weight you are lifting.
4. Cool down. You can repeat the warm up exercise but do it slower than during the warm up.
5. Stretch after any set of strengthening exercises. This prevents your muscles from becoming tight.
6. Be consistent. Stay on a regular schedule throughout the work day and work week.
7. Forget all about "No Pain, No Gain." Any strengthening exercise that causes pain should be stopped or changed! It is normal to feel some soreness two or three days after starting new strengthening exercises. The soreness should get better after three to four days.

Nervie and Disco became excited to start their exercise program. They began competing against each other and wanted to see who was stronger. They approached their workout leader once again.

Nervie & Disco: How can we check our leg strength?

Sergio then demonstrated to them how to check their leg strength. But he warned them: Any body part that is or gets noticeably weaker, even with exercises, should be looked at by a medical professional, especially if you also have pain.

Sergio: Stand up on your toes. Can you do it on one foot? Is the right side the same as on the left?

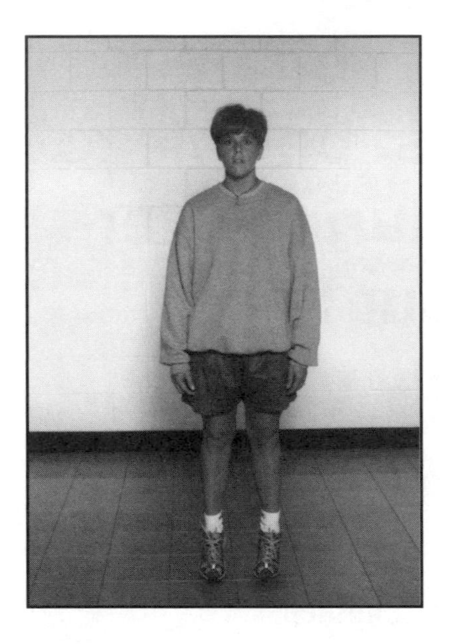

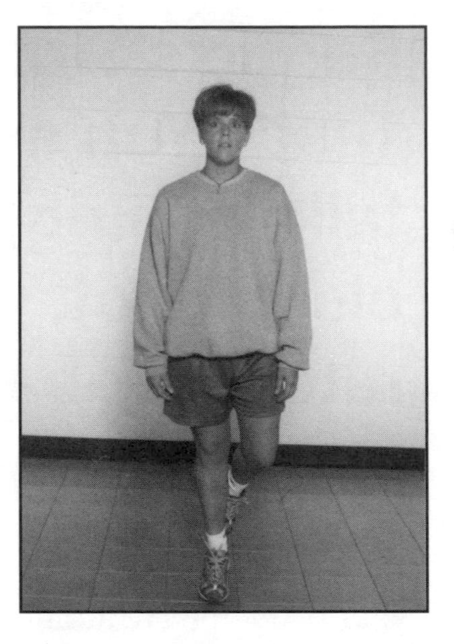

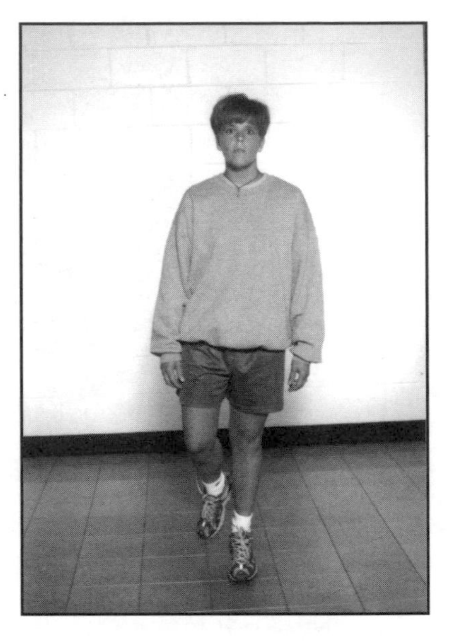

Sergio: Now squat down. Do this in front of a mirror. See if you lean to one side? Can you place the same amount of weight on the right and left leg? How does it compare to the last time? This tests the general strength of your legs.

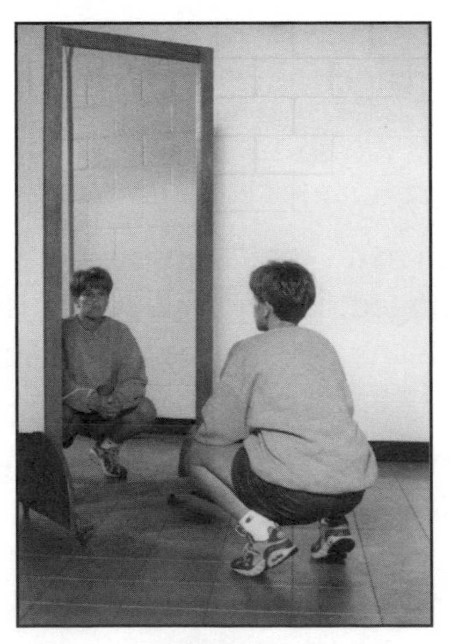

Sergio: The previous two exercises are a quick way to check your leg strength. The more times you can repeat each one, the stronger you are. You can check your progress periodically by repeating these tests.

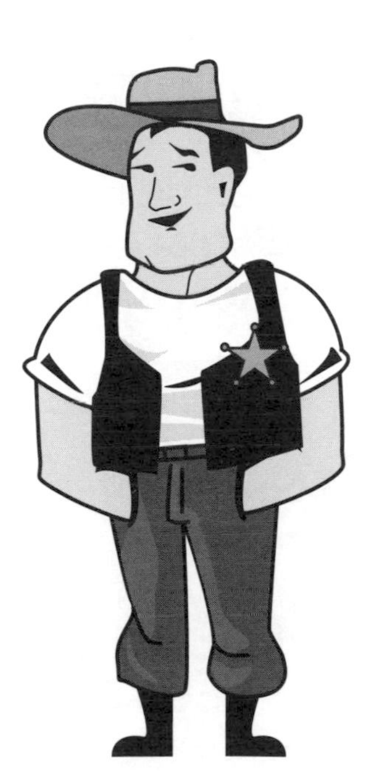

Sergio's Tip: You are never too young to start exercising.

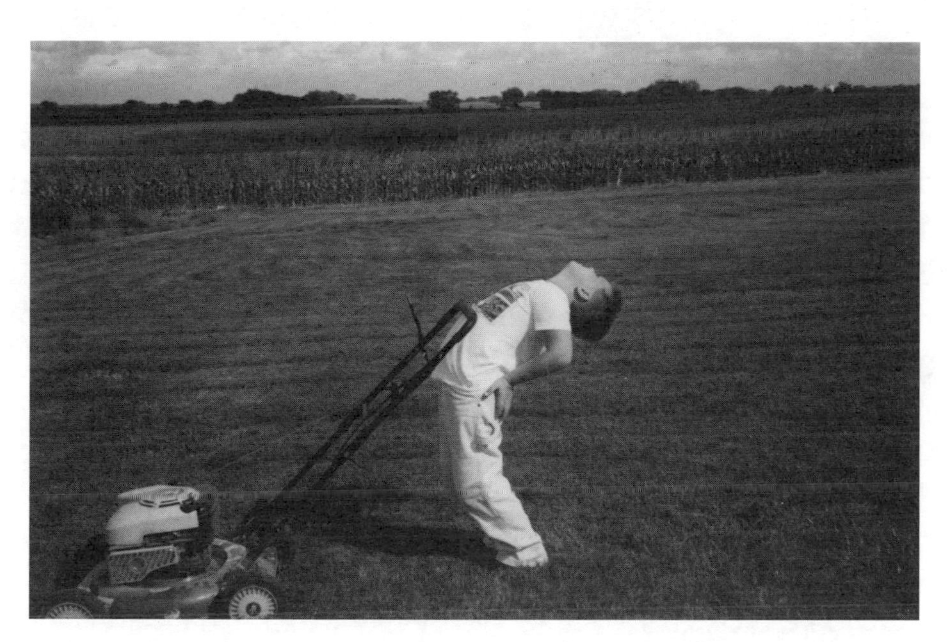

Chapter 3

Disco's Story: How do Your Discs Work?

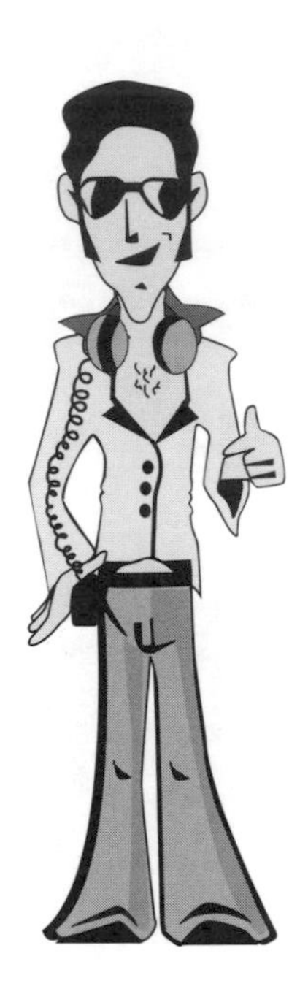

Disco loves to dance. His favorite dance move is the forward roll, a popular move from the 70s. Whenever he danced, Disco performed the forward roll over and over again. Little did he know this move put stress on the discs of his lower back. When he was younger, he had no problems with bending or twisting his back. Now that he is a bit older and he works many hours, things are different.

Disco worksas a manual laborer, and does a lot of lifting, twisting and turning. Disco never bent his knees during lifting, and he always worked with his body bent forward. This along with his dancing, put too much stress on the discs in his lower back. Sergio would constantly remind Disco to work smarter but his words fell on Disco's deaf ears.

One day it finally happened. Disco bent forward to lift a computer and felt a sharp pain in his back and leg. Disco, became concerned and quickly went to see the doctor. Luckily, he did not need surgery. His doctor told him that if he does the right exercises and worked smarter, his pain will eventually go away. Disco, now more than ever, began to listen to Sergio's advice. He also started to pay more attention to his daily behaviors. He went to a physical therapist who taught him what exercises to do and how to work smarter. Disco was soon pain-free.

Disco's recovery made him very interested in how he got his pain. He wanted to understand how exercise cured him. After careful research, he found that the answer was in how the discs of the back work.

Disco started his research by looking up disc problems on the Internet. *Herniated, ruptured, and bulging* discs are just a few of the terms he found. To better understand, he downloaded diagrams that showed what each of these disc problems look like.

Conceptual Model of the Disc

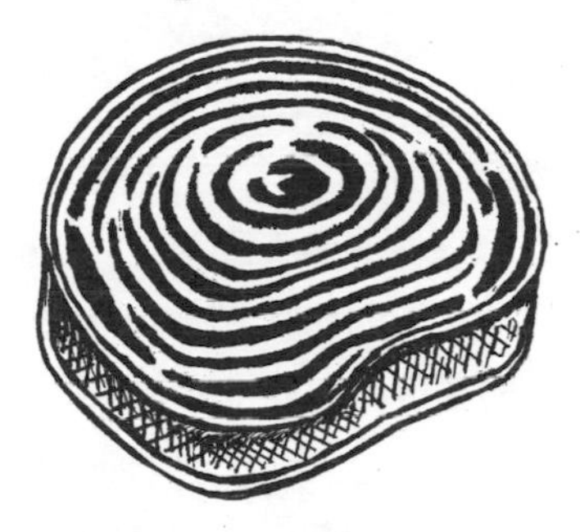

A normal disc has its fluid evenly distributed inside the disc.

Normal Disc

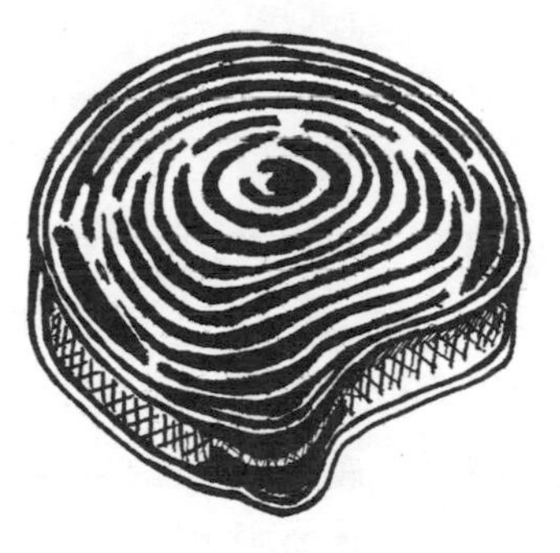

A bulging disc has its fluid pushing against one side of the disc wall. The fluid remains inside the disc, however the fluid might cause the disc wall to bulge far enough to press on a nerve nearby.

Bulging Disc

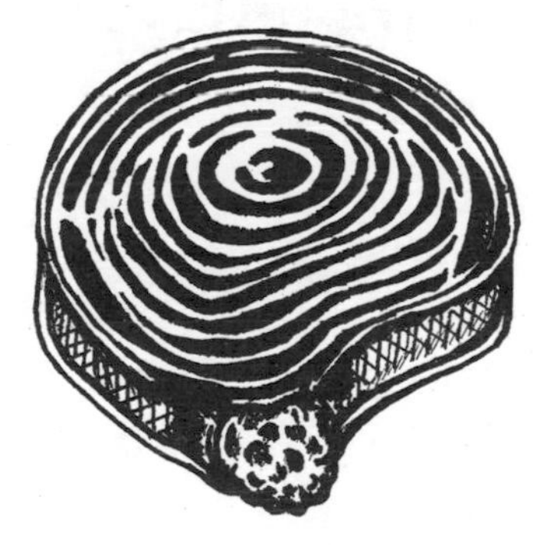

A herniated disc has its fluid escape through a disc wall. This fluid remains outside the disc and can easily press on a nerve nearby.

Herniated or Ruptured Disc

Disco learned that there are many ways to treat disc conditions. Disco learned how different movements affected discs. He learned that too much forward bending was harmful to the spine and that he needed to balance the forward bending with backward bending.

The next day he went to work and picked Sergio's brain.

Disco: What happens to your discs when you bend forward at the waist?

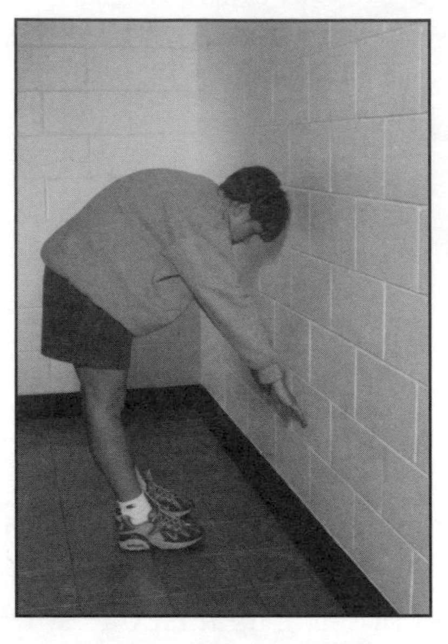

back of body

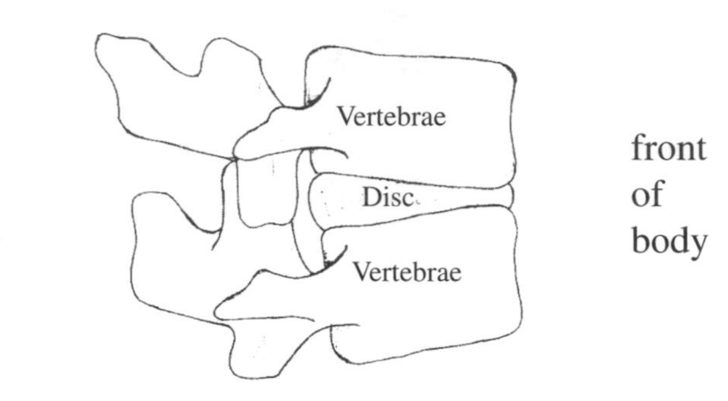

front of body

Sergio: When you sit, wash your hands, drive, eat, watch TV or pick up objects, you bend forward, placing your spine in a forward bent position. Forward bending is a more common activity than backward bending. Forward bending applies pressure to the front of your discs. This pressure pushes the fluid to the back of the discs, which can cause the discs to lose their normal shape. When the discs change shape they can cause pain.

Disco: This makes sense but what happens when you bend backward?

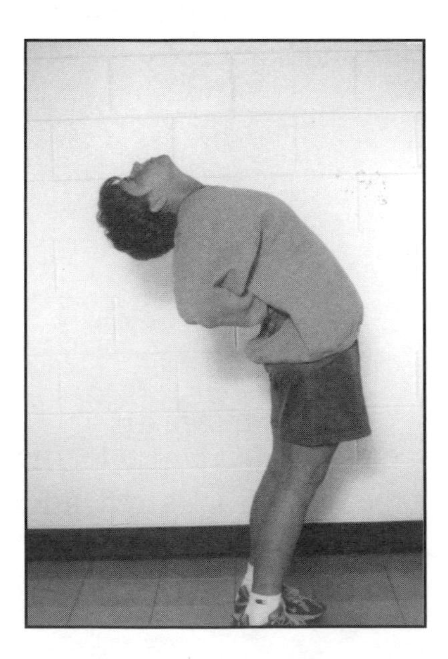

back of body

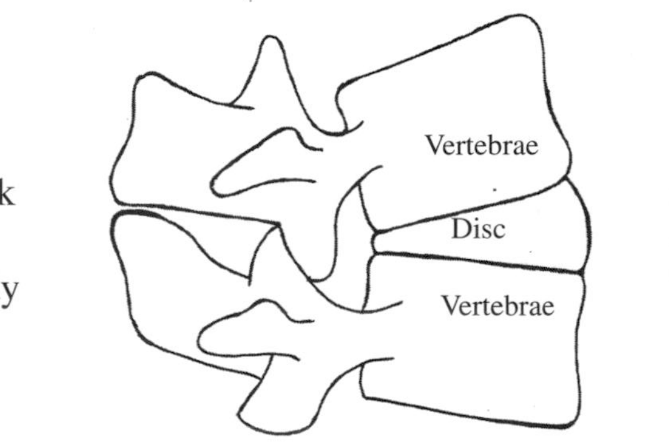

front of body

Sergio: Backward bending applies pressure to the back of your discs. This pressure pushes the fluid to the front of the discs. People who sit or bend very often can help keep their discs normal by performing a back bending exercise. This conteracts the many times of the day that we forward bend.

Disco: How am I supposed to know what is an awkward position for my spine and what is normal?

Sergio: Everyone bends and twists in awkward positions. However, a spine that has a normal curve is less likely to become injured.

Disco: How do I know whether my spine has a normal curve?

Sergio: This is how you look with a normal lower back curve.

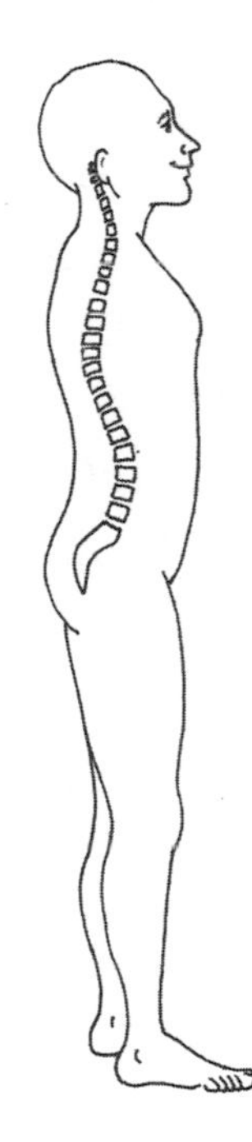

The spine has three natural curves that allow for mobility and flexibility. The curve in your lower back is called your lumbar lordosis.

Sergio: This is how you look with an increased lower back curve.

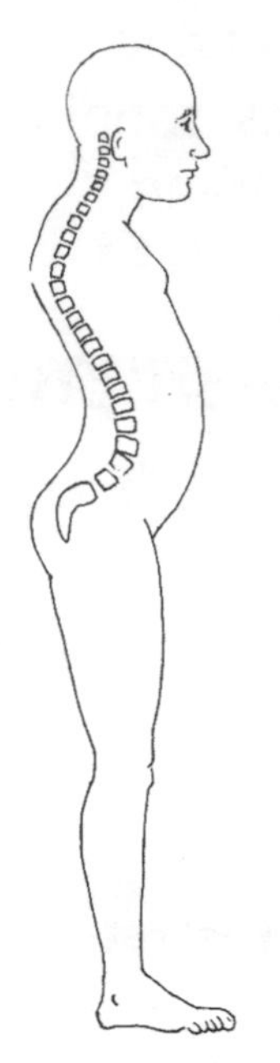

When the lower back curve is increased, you have a "sway back". If you have sway back, the joints in your lower back are closer in proximity than they should be and will likely cause abnormal stress on the lower back structures. Tight thigh muscles in the front of your legs (quadriceps) or weak abdominal muscles can cause sway back. You can maintain a pain free spine by performing the stretches and strengthening exercises that compensate for the sway back. Exercises such as bilateral knees to chest, squatting and sit ups are just some of the examples. (See exercises on pages 39-41, 44)

Sergio: This is how you look with a decreased lower back curve.

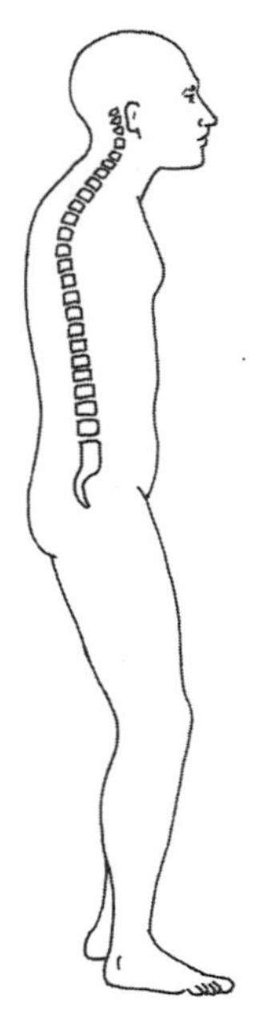

When the lower back curve is decreased, you have a "flat back". If you have a flat back, the joints in your lower back are further in proximity than they should be and will likely cause abnormal stress on the lower back structures. Tight muscles in the back of your legs (hamstrings) decreases the curve in your lower back and causes flat back. You can perform prone press up exercises to maintain your spine flexibility. (See exercises on page 26 and 27).

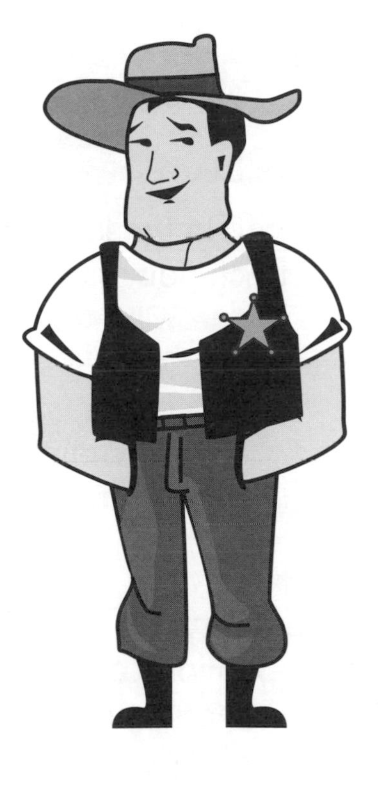

Sergio's Tip: If you are currently feeling pain in your lower back, stand up and roll your pelvis forward and backward, trying to find the most comfortable and pain-free position for your pelvis. Once you find that position, try and maintain it 30-60 seconds every hour of the day.

Disco: Why did I feel pain when I woke up this morning?

Sergio: There are many reasons you felt pain when you woke up this morning. Here is one of them.

Your discs went out drinking while you were sleeping.

Normal body fluid enters the discs when you sleep at night. In fact, people are taller in the morning for this very reason. The reason the discs "drink" this fluid is that it is full of healthy vitamins and minerals. That is how the discs stay healthy. When you stand up for the first time in the morning, the body puts all of its weight on the discs. This forces the excess fluid to leave the discs. It takes a while to do this. If you twist or bend on a full disc, it may be too much for the disc to handle and you can end up with pain. Instead of the fluid staying in the center of the disc, the fluid will be pushed toward one side of the disc wall. If the disc wall is intact and the fluid does not escape outside of the disc a **bulging disc occurs**. A **herniated disc** is one step worse than a bulging disc. A herniated disc is when the fluid escapes and breaks through the disc wall. Both a bulging and a herniated disc can cause pain. Pain is caused when a nerve is irritated either from something pressing on it or from inflammation. What adds to the problem is that we have to bend forward to wash up, dress, put our shoes on, sit and so on. So our discs are stressed throughout the day as well.

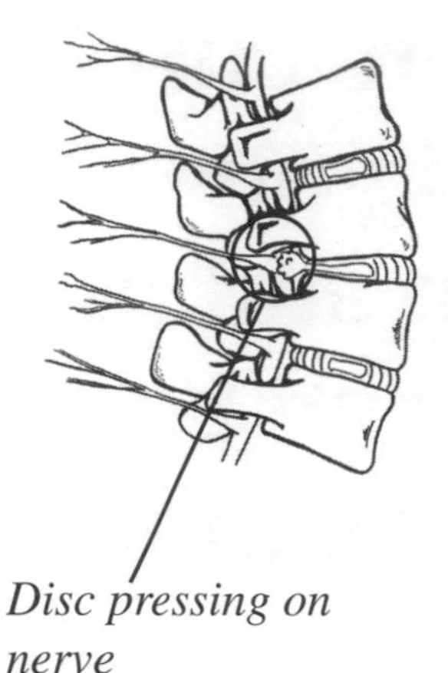

Disc pressing on nerve

What a Bulging or Herniated Disc Feels Like:

Usually one would feel numbness anywhere in the leg with or without pain. There may not be much back pain or stiffness.

What to Do:

There is a simple solution to counteract the effects of frequent forward bending on a full disc. Ideally, first thing in the morning, perform 10 repetitions of extension in a lying position (prone press ups on page 27). This should be done before you even get out of bed. Repeated extension exercises will pump out some of the fluid from the disc and will allow you to move with less risk of pain. If you have trouble doing this exercise because of pain elsewhere such as your neck, shoulder or arms, try standing back bends.

Sergio: Disco, these are the exercises you should do every morning when you get up.

The following three exercises stretch the front of the spine.

Elbow Rest (This exercise is also a great afternoon or evening exercise to counteract long periods of sitting).

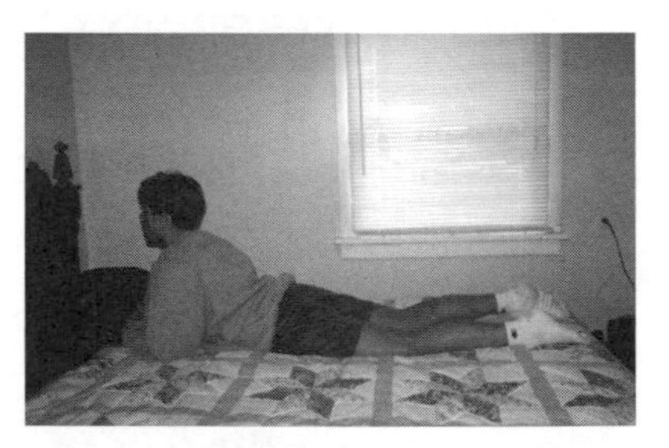

Purpose: To extend the lower back

- Lie on your stomach while resting on your elbows.
- Let your hips and abdomen sag (relax) on the floor or bed.

This is a good resting position and should be sustained for one minute if it does not cause pain.

Prone Press Ups

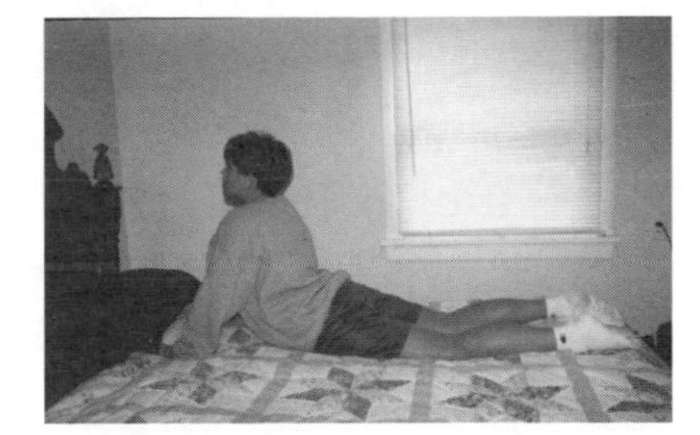

Purpose: To extend the lower back (counteract constant sitting). This exercise can be attempted if the Elbow Rest is comfortable.

- Lie on the floor face down with your hands flat on the floor by your shoulders.
- Press up on your hands and try to sustain your body weight on your arms while relaxing your hips and back muscles.

Hold for one second and repeat 10 times. This can be repeated many times during the day to counteract the forward bending postures.

Standing Back Bends

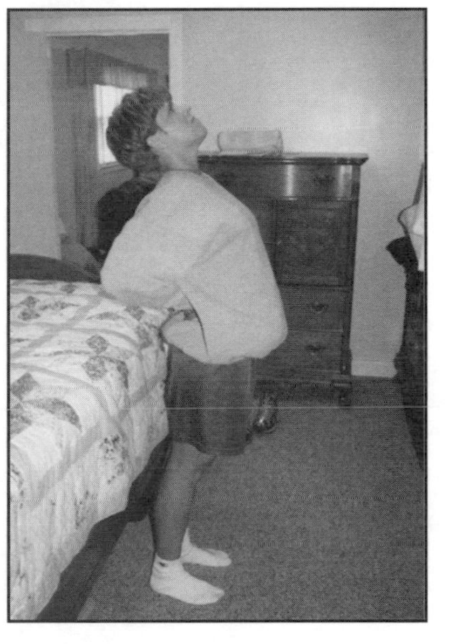

This should be done only if the Prone Press Ups are too uncomfortable.

Purpose: To take pressure off the back of your discs and stretch the front ligaments and muscles.

- Stand with your feet shoulder width apart.
- You may want to stand with your back against a kitchen counter or a sturdy object that does not reach above your buttocks.
- Place your hands on the middle of your lower back.
- Leading with your head, lean back as far as possible. Keep your knees straight during the entire exercise.

Hold for 1 second and repeat 10 times. This can be repeated many times during the day to counteract the forward bending postures.

Bilateral Knee to Chest

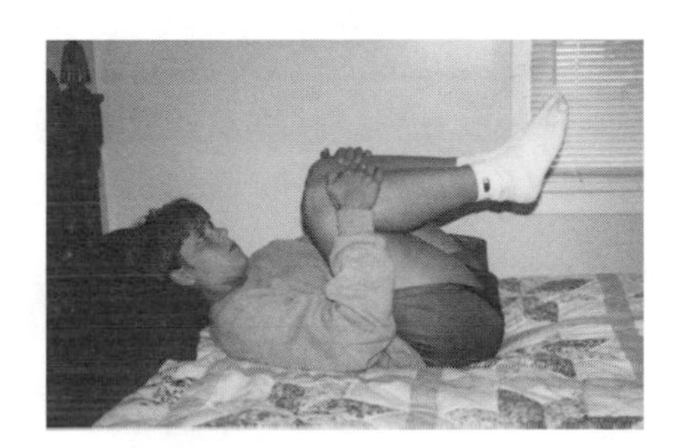

Purpose: To stretch the lower back muscles.

- Lie on your back with your knees bent and your feet flat on the floor.
- Bring both knees toward your chest and grab them with your hands just below the knee.

Hold for 20 seconds and return slowly to the starting position.

Piriformis Stretch

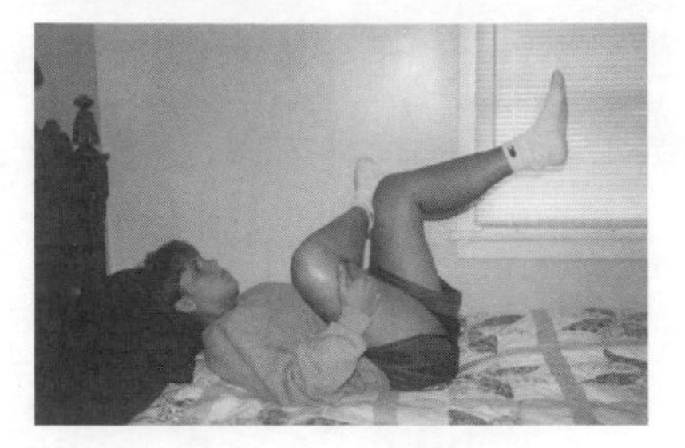

Purpose: To stretch the piriformis muscle, which will take pressure off the sciatic nerve.

- Lie on your back with your knees bent.
- Cross your right leg over your left leg above your knee.
- Clasp your right hand behind your right knee and your left hand behind your left knee. Bring your legs toward your chest.

Hold for 20 seconds and repeat on the right side. You should feel a stretching sensation in the buttock.

Now try the following exercise:

Sit on a bed or chair relaxed and slouched.

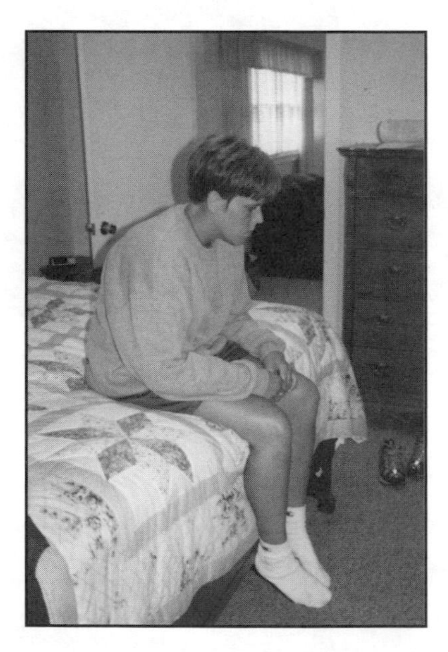

Then sit as tall as you can and place your hand in the small curve of your back.

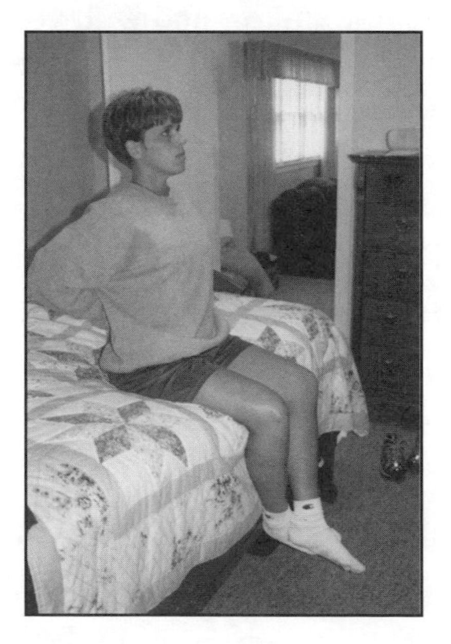

This is a great exercise to do when sitting for long periods of time. It helps improve your sitting posture and is inconspicuous and not time-consuming.

Chapter 4

Nervie's Story: How Your Nerves Work.

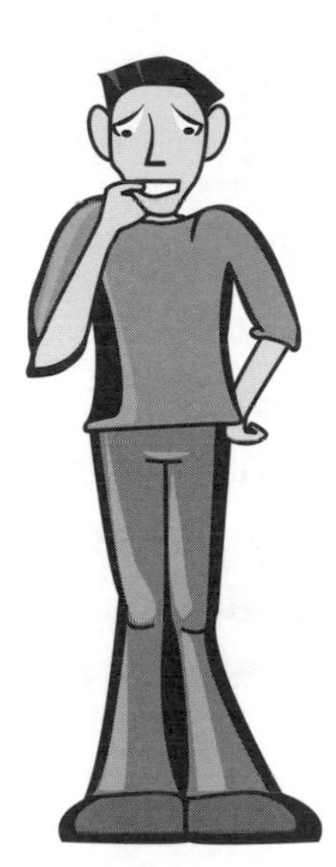

Nervie could talk for hours on end. The muscles of his mouth were in great shape, but the rest of his body wasn't. Often, he would sit slouched in front of his computer typing and chatting on line. He also worried about everything, which caused him to smoke, his muscles to tense up and his posture to slump forward. Nervie was a chain-smoking, malnourished, out-of-shape computer worker who never exercised.

Little did Nervie know that his stressful lifestyle was causing his back and neck muscles to tense up. The muscles in his lower back became extremely tight and began to press on his sciatic nerve. This resulted in a shooting pain from his lower back to his foot. His slumped forward posture caused his disc fluid to bulge in one direction. The bulging disc in his lower back started to press on his sciatic nerve, causing further pain and discomfort.

Unfortunately for his co-workers and friends, Nervie's last good nerve was the one stretching to his mouth. Why wasn't this nerve pressed on to cause his mouth to hurt? The answer was simple. Nervie exercised his mouth. He soon realized that if he could exercise the rest of his body as well, his back and neck pain might go away. Nervie decided that he needed to take other steps to correct his aches and pains as well. He stopped smoking and became more concerned about his posture. He made an effort to sit and stand up straight. Nervie's pain started to go away, and his overall disposition improved. His body hurt less, and he stopped worrying so much, which made him more bearable to be around.

Nervie became increasingly interested in how his nerves worked and wanted to avoid a repeat of the pain he had felt. He studied the human body and was taught by Sergio how to preserve the health of the nerves exiting his spine. Nervie was excited about his new found knowledge. He now talks Sergio's ear off, asking him questions about ergonomics and lower back health.

Nervie: Sergio, how do my nerves work?

Sergio: Nerves are responsible for sending information to muscles to carry out movement, interpret sensation and protect us by monitoring our systems and our surroundings. Healthy nerves exit our spinal cord and attach themselves to the structures they are monitoring. When the nerves are pinched on, they send us an unpleasant message of pain. A tight muscle, a poorly aligned spine, a herniated or bulging disc, or an inflamed joint can all pinch on a nerve.

Nervie: My doctor told me I had sciatica. He said my sciatic nerve was being pressed on. How did this happen?

Sergio: This is what happens when your sciatic nerve gets pressed on. The sciatic is a group of nerves that run from your lower back down to your toes. A herniated or bulging disc, or inflamed joints in the back may press on it, causing shooting pain, tingling or numbness from the back or buttocks down the leg. The piriformis muscle, which is located in the buttock, can also press on the sciatic nerve to produce these same sensations.

Nervie: How can you avoid getting sciatica?

Sergio: You can help avoid sciatica with this stretch:

Piriformis Stretch

Purpose: To stretch the piriformis muscle, which will take pressure off the sciatic nerve.

- Lie on your back with your knees bent.
- Cross your right leg over your left leg above your knee.
- Clasp your right hand behind your right knee and your left hand behind your left knee. Bring your legs toward your chest.

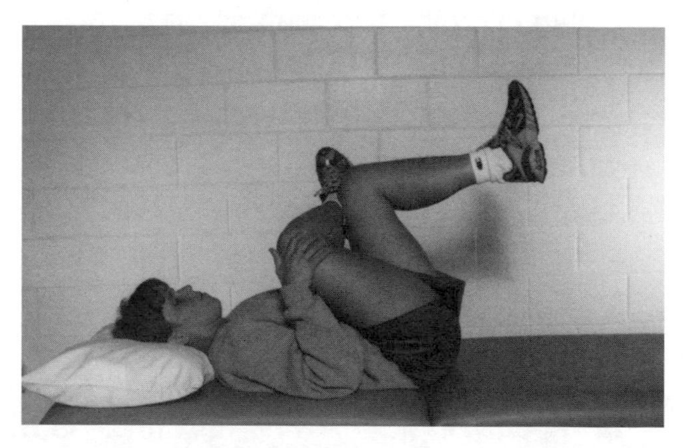

Hold for 20 seconds and repeat on the left side. You should feel a stretching sensation in the buttock.

Sitting Piriformis Sretch

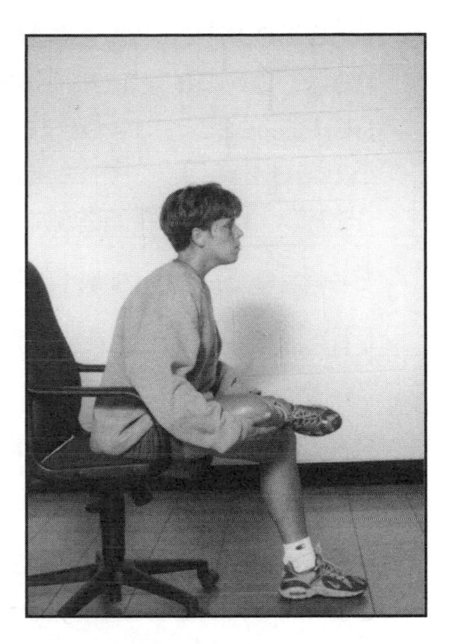

Purpose: To stretch the piriformis muscle, which will take pressure off the sciatic nerve.

- Place both feet flat on the ground.
- Lift your right foot up and place it on your left knee.
- Lean forward slowly, being careful not to lose your balance.

Hold for 20 seconds and repeat on the left side. You should feel a stretching sensation in the buttock.

Nervie: Why did my Physical Therapist treat my back when I had a shooting pain down my legs?

Sergio: This is a very common question asked by many who suffer from back pain. The answer is referred pain. By definition, referred pain is pain that is felt at a location other than the actual problem area. You might experience pain and numbness down your leg into your foot. Is the problem area in your foot or is it in your back? Nerves exiting your spinal cord in your lower back travel all the way down to your toes. If you have a pinched nerve in your back, you may feel pain anywhere that the nerve travels, including your lower legs, yet feel no back pain. The pain you feel could be only in your legs, only in your back, or both. A telltale sign that your back problem is getting worse is when pain intensifies further down your legs. Conversely, if your leg pain is improving your back problem is probably improving.

Nervie: At one time my leg felt numb even though my back pain was gone. Why did this happen?

Sergio: This is why it happens:

Most people who get medical treatment for back pain get better within two or three months. It is common to have no pain but still have some numbness in the leg. That's because the parts of the back that produced the back pain are different from the parts that cause the numbness. These different parts may take different time to heal.

People who have had back and leg pain for many months may have injured a nerve in the back. Since the nerves from the back travel down to the leg, the numbness may be felt anywhere the nerve travels. A damaged nerve may cause the numbness in your legs. The good news is that the nerve can heal itself. The bad news is that it takes months to heal.

Sergio: This is what nerve damage feels like:

There is numbness anywhere in the leg with or without pain. There is usually no back pain or stiffness.

Sergio: This is what you should do about the numbness.

First you should see if the numbness gets worse with time. You can do this by rating it each week. Give your numbness a number from 1 to 10 and write it down. If the numbness gets worse, a specialist should examine you. A physiatrist (a rehabilitation doctor), a neurologist, orthopedist, or your family doctor can perform special tests for the nerves. It is not unusual for the numbness to take months or even a year to completely disappear. If the numbness does not interfere with your everyday activities and it is not worsening, then it is generally not harmful. If there is any doubt, see your family doctor for advice.

When we develop pain or numbness, we have a tendency to reduce our activities. This may lead to general stiffness. Here is an easy way to check for general stiffness.

Start by facing a wall standing two-foot lengths away. Bend forward and try to let your hands touch the lowest part of the wall. Mark the spot that both hands touch the wall. Perform this motion every 2 or 3 days and compare the marks on the wall.

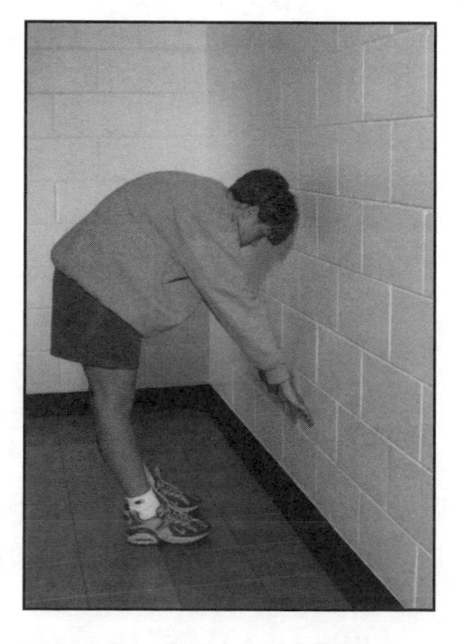

Now stand with your feet shoulder width apart and your hands on the small of your back. Bend back as far as you can and look at the lowest spot on the wall. Compare this spot to the next time you do this. When doing these exercises, you may feel a tightness, pressure or pain in the back, but it should go away once you stop and stand up straight.

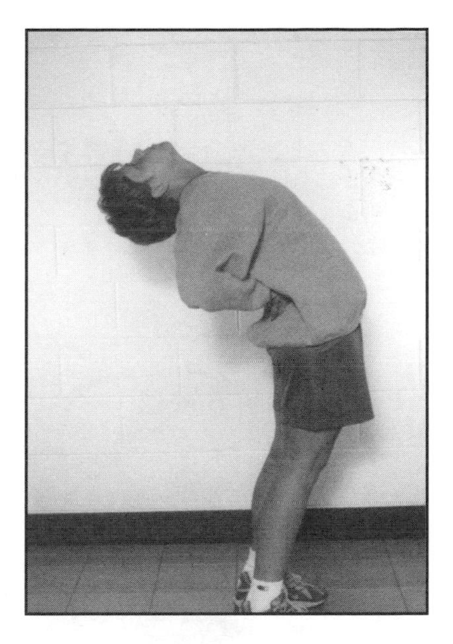

With your feet shoulder width apart, slide your hips to one side and your shoulder to the other. Turn around and do this in the opposite direction. Compare the amount of hip motion of your right side to your left side. Also compare it to the next time you do this. Both sides should feel the same.

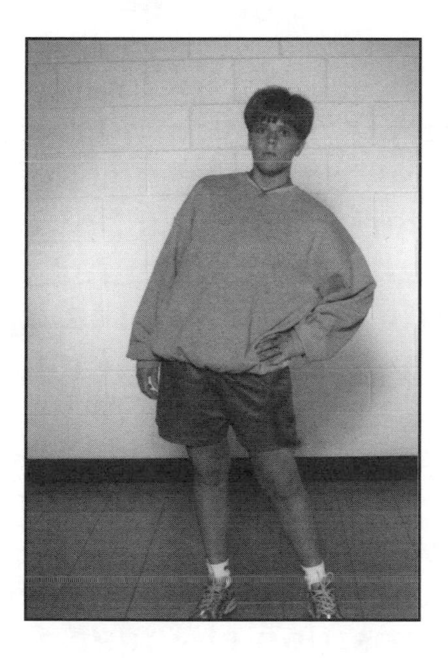

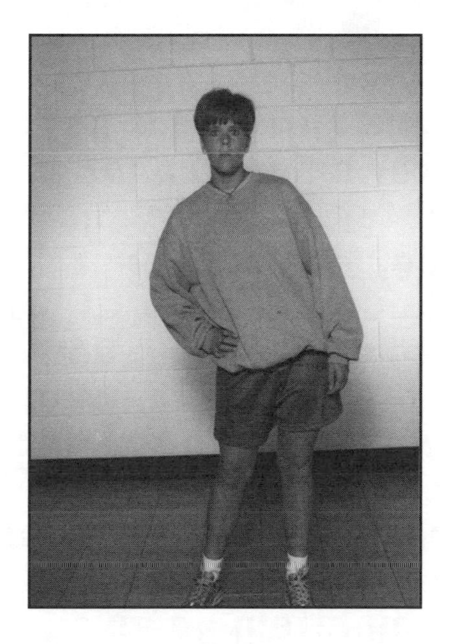

In summary, if your numbness gets worse while your back gets stiffer, you should see a medical doctor, a physical therapist or chiropractor as soon as possible.

Chapter 5

Muskull's Story: How Your Muscles Work

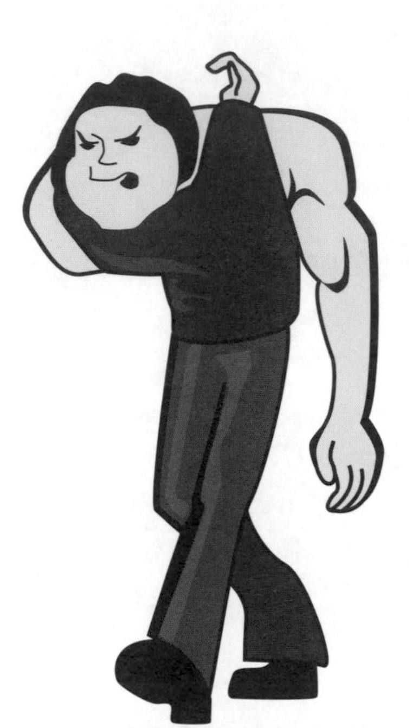

Muskull is a muscle-head. He has dedicated his life to pumping up his muscles. Muskull used to be as strong as an ox. He regularly went to the gym and always tried to lift as much weight as his muscles would allow him to. His body mechanics were poor since he emphasized how much, not how well he could lift. At first, Muskull was able to get away with this bad habit. However, as time went by, Muskull's muscles became less flexible. Though he was more prone to a muscle injury, it did not matter to Muskull because people saw how big he was not how inflexible his muscles had become.

Muskull carried his poor habits to his job. He was a manual laborer who did a lot of lifting, twisting and turning. Despite repeated advice on how to work properly from his boss Sergio, Muskull never changed his habits. He continued to workout and work at his job with little regard for the health of his body. One day it finally happened. Muskull pulled a muscle in his lower back and was in great pain. Muskull went to the doctor and received pain medication, which gave him some relief. But he still refused to listen to Sergio's advice, and trips to the doctor became more frequent. The discomfort from this muscle strain never seemed to completely go away. Muskull's disposition changed for the worse, his posture became progressively worse and his muscles started to weaken. He could no longer work out, and he became more reliant on his pain medication. Not being able to work out upset Muskull, so he finally gave in and asked Sergio for help.

Sergio: Muskull, allow me to explain how your muscles work.

Muscles give us the ability to move different parts of our body. The lower back has two types of muscles: postural muscles and lifting muscles. The postural muscles are thin and delicate. They support the spine for sitting or standing. If you maintain your posture in one position for a long period of time without change, these muscles will get tired and weak.

The lifting muscles are some of the strongest muscles in your body and are very powerful. However, if you use faulty body mechanics when lifting, you can easily strain these muscles, especially if they are fatigued. This would make you more prone to an injury.

Sergio: Here is a common muscle injury:

Muscle Strain

A muscle strain is a tear in the muscle. The tear can be extensive and can result in minor or severe pain. A muscle that is constantly at work will tend to fatigue. As a muscle becomes tired, it tightens and loses its flexibility, becoming more susceptible to injury. It will injure if it is not stretched regularly. Stretching keep muscles limber and allows blood to flow freely and nourish them. Performing stretching exercises daily, will allow your muscles to move with less risk of injury. Stretching for as little as one minute every hour will help your body move freely. That adds up to less than 10 minutes of stretching for each day.

If you use proper body mechanics during lifting, maintain good work habits and ergonomic design, you will reduce the strain placed on your muscles.

Muskull: Why did I pull a muscle in my back when I was tying my shoes?

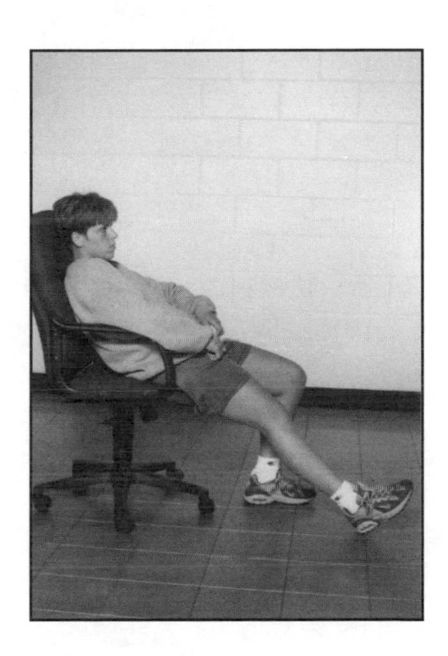

Sergio: Most people tie their shoes while sitting or standing and bending. If you think about it, sitting and bending or sitting slouched is one of the most common movements that we perform. By repeating this many times every day, sometimes 3,000-5,000 times a day, we overstretch our lower back in a forward direction.

What a muscle strain feels like: You may feel sudden sharp back pain that may be worse on one side. You may have difficulty standing up straight immediately after rising from sitting. You may also feel pain with twisting, hiking up your hip, etc.

What to do: We bend forward 3,000-5,000 times every day but rarely bend backward. What you need to do is bend backward to keep yourself **balanced.** Here is an exercise that can be done while sitting:

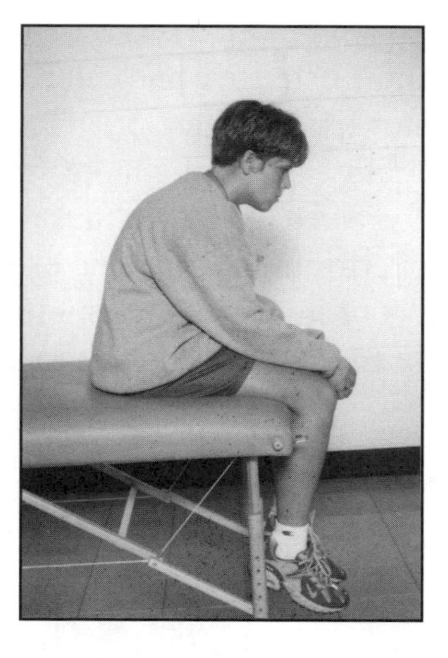

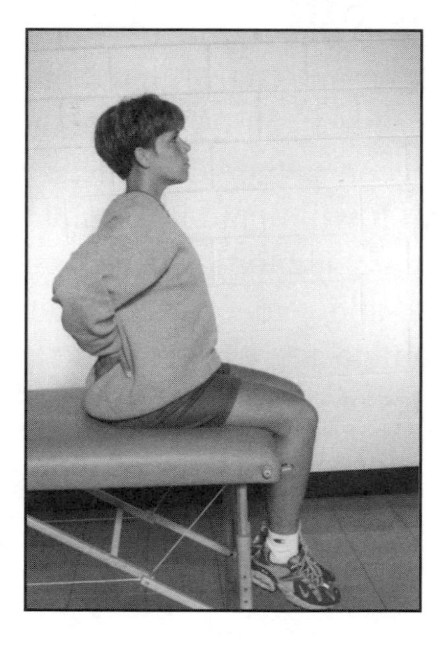

After repeating the above exercise a couple of times, you should be able to move more freely. When you can perform this movement easier and with less pain you can begin the following:

Perform this exercise for 5-10 repetitions every 2 hours for 2 days. When the pain is no longer constant, perform this exercise 3 - 4 times a day for 5-10 repetitions. As your pain decreases, you can decrease this exercise to 2 times a day for 5-10 repetitions.

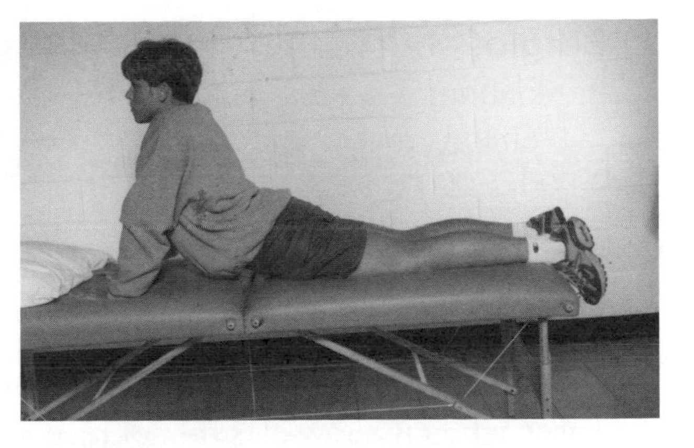

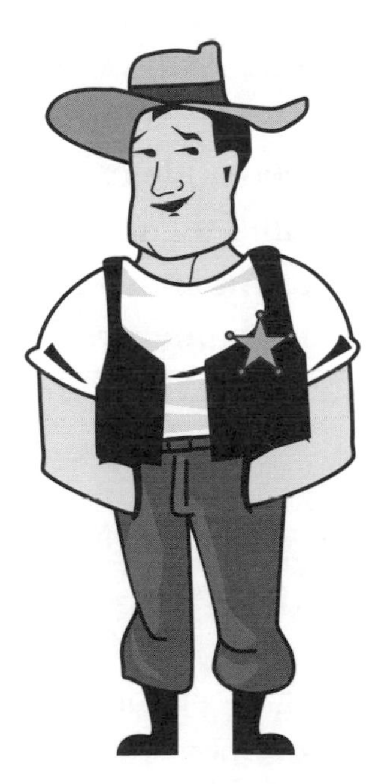

Sergio's Tip: To avoid back pain perform this exercise each morning before getting out of bed for 5 - 10 repetitions.

Muskull: Why do I get muscle spasms in my lower back?

Sergio: A muscle spasm is your body's way of telling you to slow down before you get seriously hurt. A spasm typically feels like an ache. Muscle aches prevent you from continuing a particular activity that would be harmful. This is known as "muscle guarding". A spasm is triggered when you consistently decrease the blood flow to your muscle ("decreased circulation"). When you overwork a muscle and do not provide it with sufficient rest, circulation of blood is decreased. When blood flow decreases, the waste products that the muscle produces tend to accumulate and eventually stop the muscle from working properly. This decrease in blood supply causes further loss of movement, which brings on muscle spasms and may cause further pain. The blood that flows to your muscles is similar to the oxygen you breathe. Without oxygen, your lungs will gasp for air; without rest and blood supply, your muscles will start to ache. So it is important to remember that whenever a muscle starts to spasm, you should stop what you are doing and rest. A muscle spasm is your body's way of telling you that you are overstepping safety boundaries and are risking an avoidable injury.

Muskull: Why is blood supply important?

Sergio: Blood is the fuel that keeps your muscles healthy and moving.

After a long, hard day at work, irritating waste products accumulate in the muscles. Ideally, your blood supply flushes out these irritating waste products, bringing the necessary vitamins and minerals to help repair and refuel the muscles. A problem arises when the muscles do not receive sufficient blood. The muscles tense up and muscle soreness occurs. Muscle soreness even occurs in well-trained athletes whose job it is to exercise all day. However, well-trained athletes understand the importance of stretching and resting their muscles after exercise. Resting gives the muscles time to repair, while stretching increases the blood supply to the muscles being stretched. Athletes understand that the more you stretch and rest, the greater you will perform.

The working person is similar to an athlete. The worker develops fatigued muscles as the working day progresses. However, when a worker takes a rest period, he or she usually sits for several minutes, which keeps the spine in a flexed posture. If you perform sitting activities or lifting activities all day, then the sitting "rest" doesn't really provide rest to your spine. You are still flexing your spine and not allowing the muscles to rest. A worker who sits and flexes his or her spine all day needs to bend backward throughout the day to reverse the flexed posture. We will discuss this in more detail in chapter 6 on posture.

Muskull: What can I do to increase my blood supply?

Sergio: Exercise, Exercise, Exercise!

There are many ways to increase blood supply to your muscles. Periodic stretching breaks, concentrating on good posture and proper work habits, are the most effective ways of maintaining a healthy blood flow to your muscles. Exercise and conditioning will also help your body become more efficient and less prone to fatigue and injury. A few minutes of general activities every day like the ones listed on the following pages should be enough to keep your back healthy.

Bilateral Knee to Chest

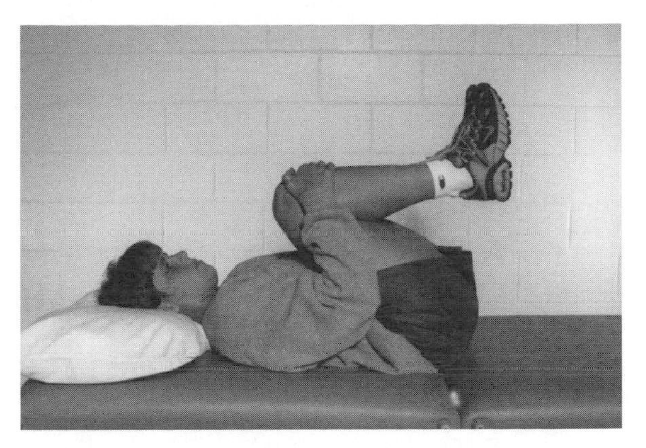

Purpose: To stretch the lower back muscles.

- Lie on your back with your knees bent and your feet flat on the floor.
- Bring both knees toward your chest and grab them with your hands just below your knees.

Hold for at least 20 seconds. Repeat once or twice.

Single Knee to Chest

Purpose: To stretch the lower back muscles on one side of your lower back.

- Lie on your back with your legs straight.
- Bring your right knee in toward your chest. (If you have knee pain, grab the back of the thigh instead of the top of the knee).

Hold for at least 20 seconds and repeat with the left leg.

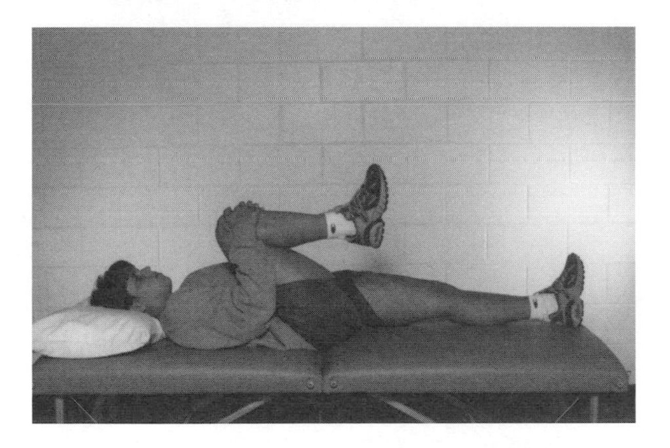

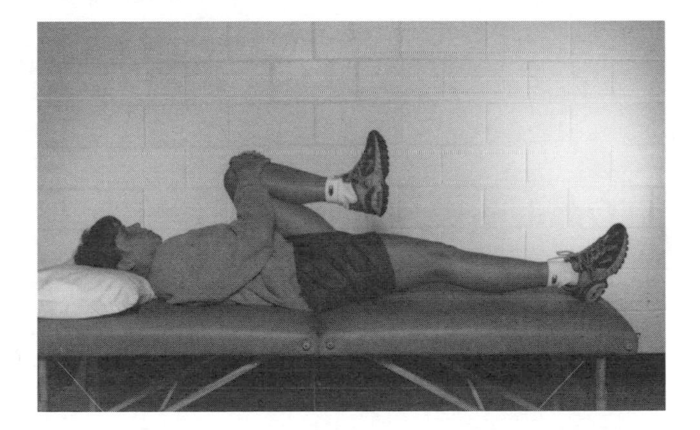

Hurdler's Stretch

Purpose: To stretch the back of one leg (hamstring) and the inner thigh of the other leg.

- Sit on the floor with your left leg directly in front of you flat on the ground.
- Bend your right knee and place the sole of your right foot against the left thigh.
- **KEEP YOUR BACK STRAIGHT** and lean forward from the hips until you feel a stretch in your hamstring (back of the leg).
- In this position you will be stretching your left hamstring.

Hold for at least 20 seconds and repeat with the right leg in front of you.

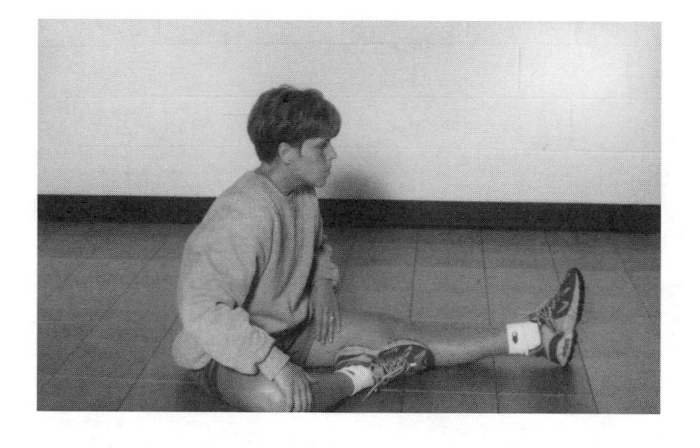

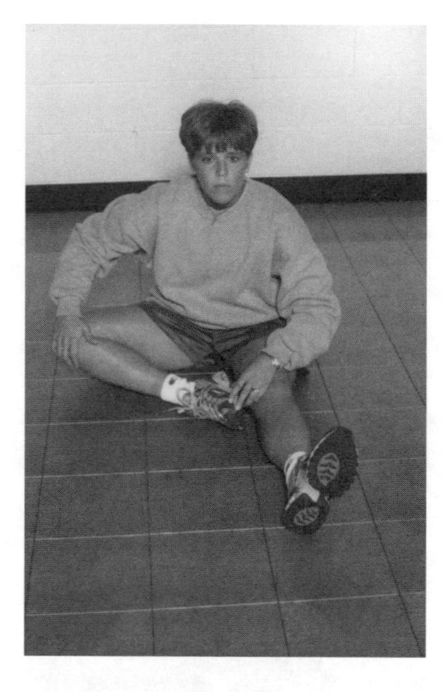

Quadriceps Stretch

Purpose: To stretch the quadricep muscles located in the front of the thigh.

Choose one of the following 3 positions.

Lying down

- Lie on your stomach and bend your left knee.
- Grab your left ankle with your left hand and bring the ankle to your buttock.

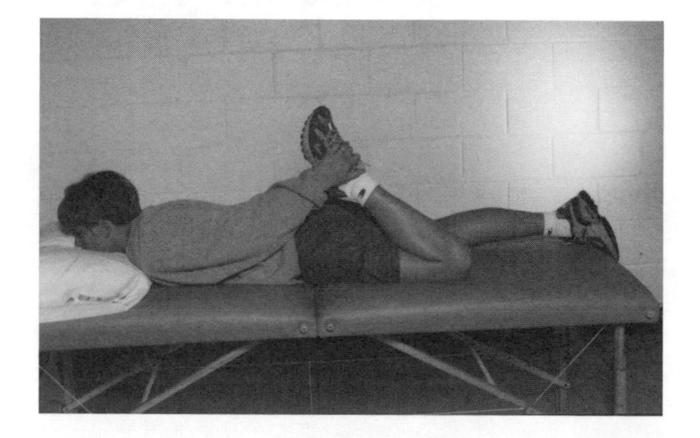

Hold for at least 20 seconds and repeat on the right side.

Sidelying - This position can be used when lying face down is not possible.

- Lie on your right side and grab your left leg right above your left ankle.
- Bend your knee back with your left hand so that your left heel is touching your buttock.

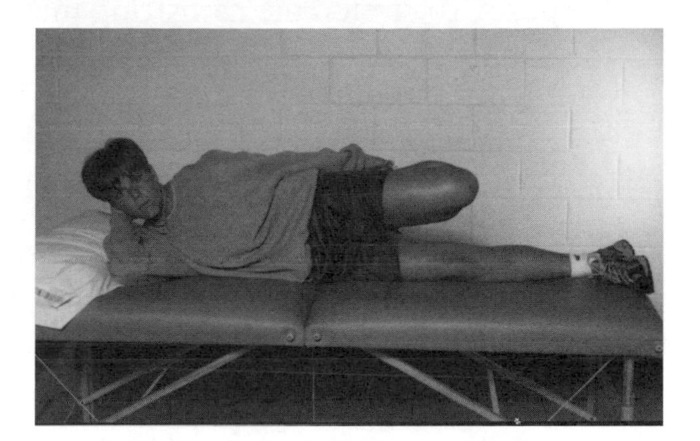

Hold for at least 20 seconds and repeat on the right side.

Standing - This position can be used as an alternative to the previous 2 exercises.

- Place your right hand on a table for support, and grab right above your left ankle with your left hand.
- With your left hand, help bend your knee bringing your heel to your buttock.

Hold for at least 20 seconds and repeat on the right side.

Note: Make sure that the knees stay close together during the entire exercise. Do not pull the thigh backward or outward.

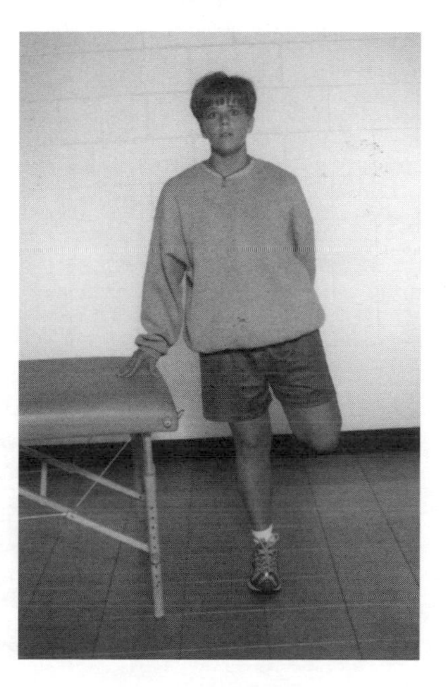

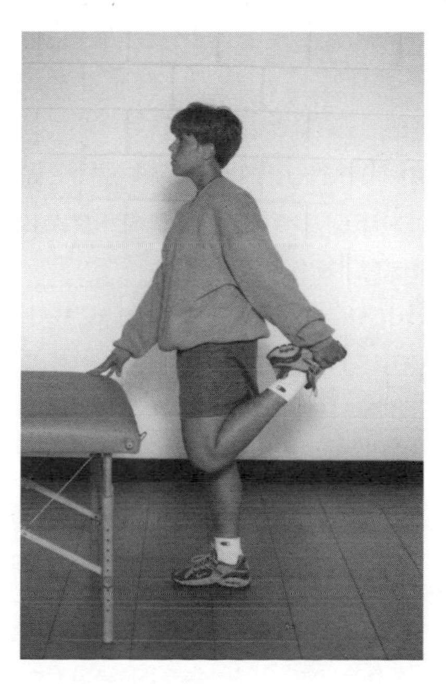

Hamstring Stretch

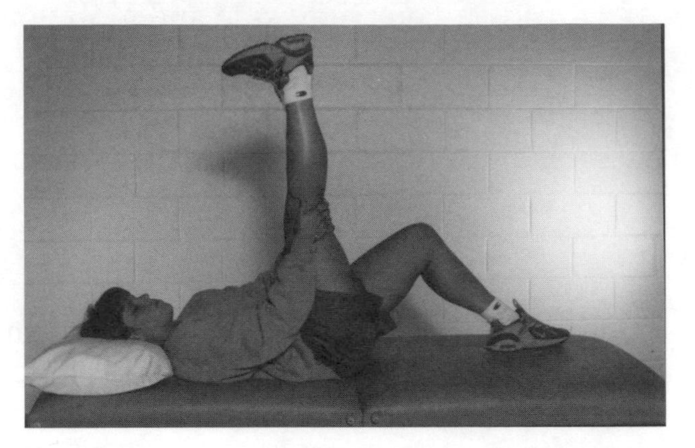

Purpose: To stretch the hamstring muscles located in the back of your thigh. Choose one of the following 3 positions.

Lying Down

- While lying on your back, clasp both hands on the back of your right thigh and lift your right leg straight up.
- Straighten your right knee.
- Point your toes toward your nose.

Hold for at least 20 seconds and repeat on the left side.

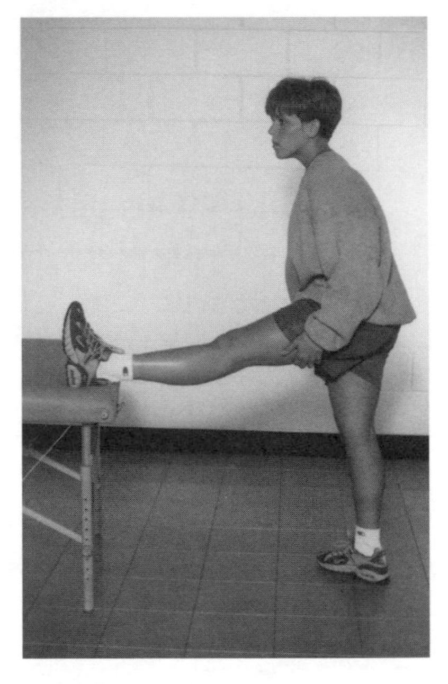

Standing Position

- While standing, place your left leg on a chair or table and keep your leg straight.
- Stand up straight and try to bring your chest to your knee.
- Keep your head straight up and make sure not to round your back.
- You should feel a comfortable pull on the left leg.

Hold for at least 20 seconds and repeat on the right side.

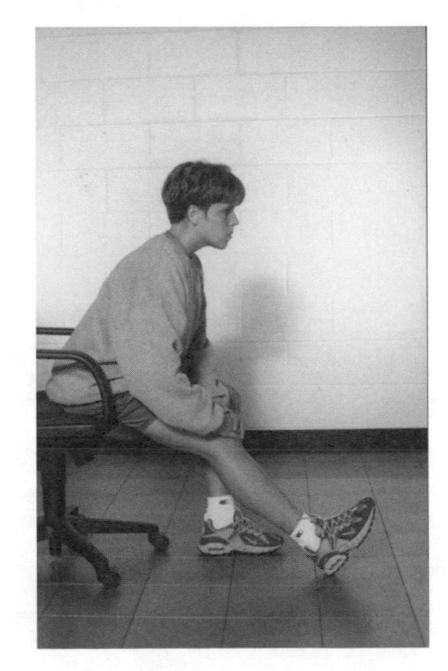

Sitting Position

Sit on the front edge of the chair.

- Bring your right leg straight out and keep your left knee bent.
- Bend forward at the waist while keeping the arch in your lower back. Do not round your shoulders forward. You should feel a stretch in the back of the leg (hamstrings).

Hold for at least 20 seconds and repeat on the left side.

Lower Back & Buttock Stretch

Purpose: To stretch the lower back and buttock.

- Lie on your back on the floor with your arms straight out to your side at shoulders height.
- Lift your right knee up to your hip, making sure to keep both shoulders and your back on the floor.
- Cross your right leg over your left leg and across your body and toward the floor. Use your left hand to help assist your right leg. Your left leg and hip should remain flat on the floor.

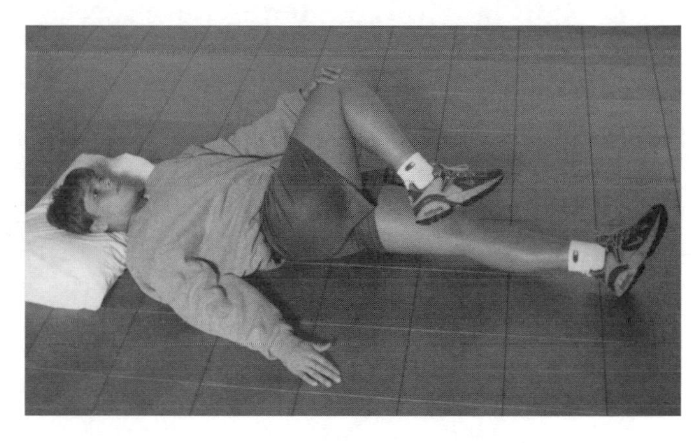

Hold for at least 20 seconds and repeat on the left side.

Pelvic Tilt

Purpose: Abdominal strengthening.

- Lie on your back with your knees bent and your feet flat on the floor.
- Place your hands behind your head.
- Press the small of your back to the floor.

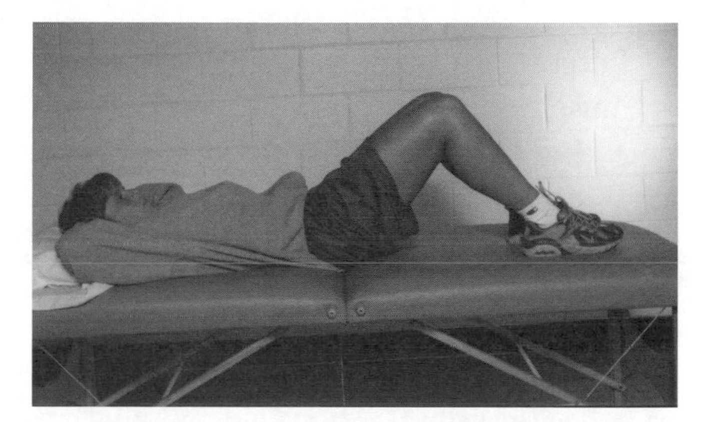

Hold for 3 seconds and repeat 10 times.

Bridging

Purpose: To strengthen the buttock and lower back muscles.

- Lie on your back with your knees bent and your feet flat on the floor.
- Lift your buttocks straight up off the floor to the ceiling while keeping your feet flat on the ground.
- Return buttocks back to the floor.

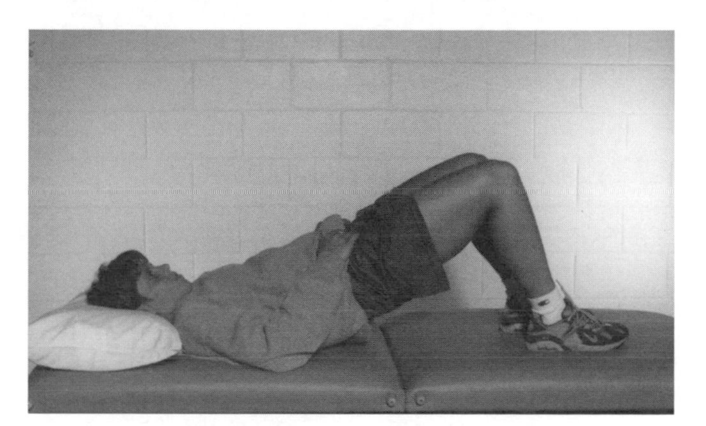

Hold buttocks in the air for 3 seconds and repeat 10 times.

Cat-Camel

Purpose: To stretch the muscles of the middle and upper back.

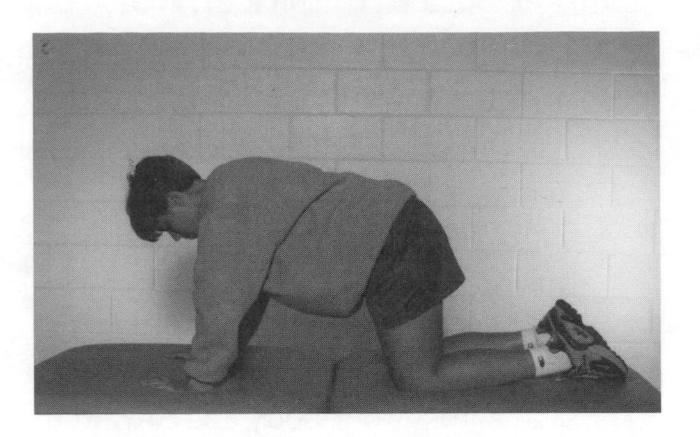

- Start on all fours, with your arms straight and your hands flat on the table. Bend knees on the table at approximately 90 degrees.
- Like an angry cat raise the middle of your back to the ceiling.
- Then let the entire back sag to the floor.

Hold for 3 seconds and repeat 10 times.

Abdominal (Stomach) Strengthening Crunches

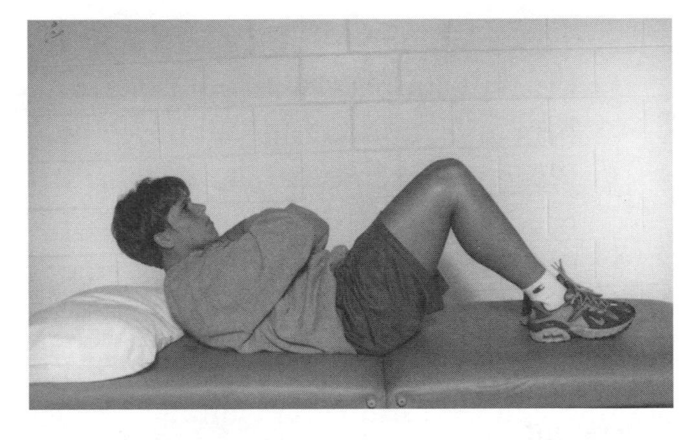

Purpose: To strengthen upper abdominal muscles.

- Lie on your back with your knees bent and your feet flat on the floor.
- Place your hands across your chest.
- Slowly raise your head and shoulders above the floor while keeping your lower and middle of your back flat against the floor. Try and get the entire shoulder blade to clear the floor.

Hold for 3 seconds and repeat 10 times.

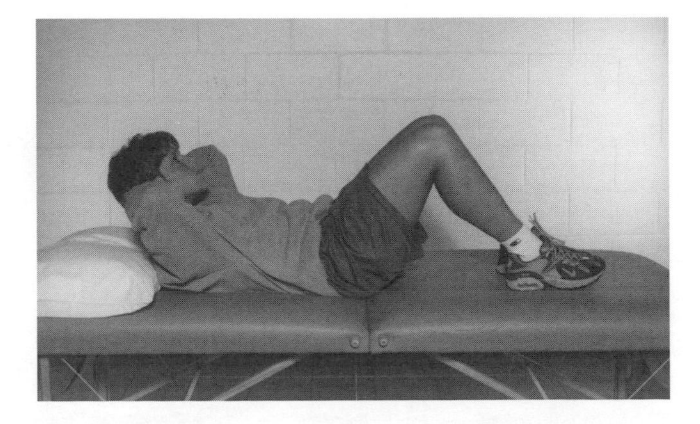

Note: The more advanced version of this exercise is done by placing your hands behind your head.

Cross-Over Crunch

Purpose: To strengthen oblique abdominal muscles along the sides of your stomach.

- Lie on your back with your knees bent.
- Place your hands behind your head.
- Lift your head and left shoulder off the floor toward your right knee.

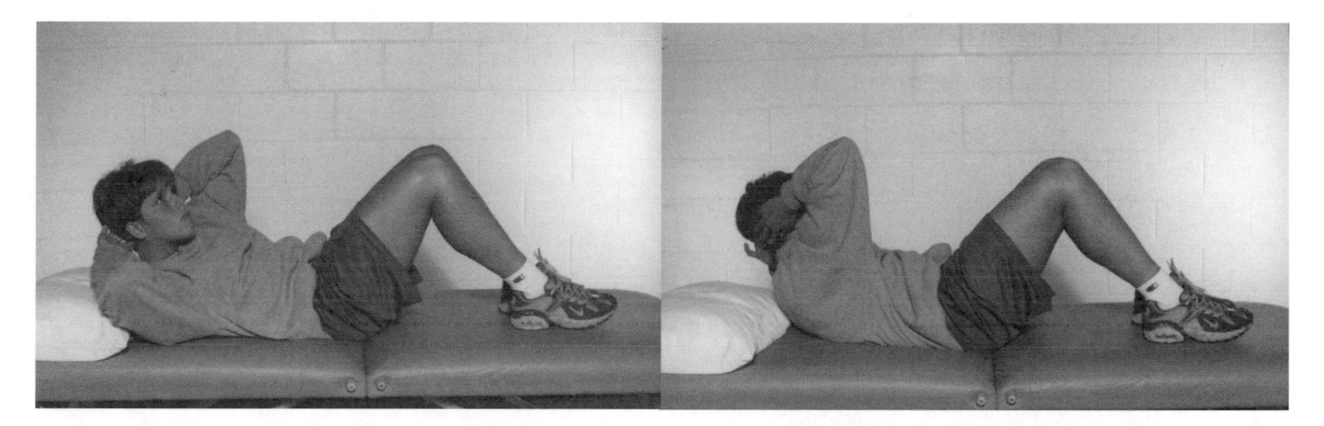

Hold this position for 3 seconds, then return to the starting position. Repeat 10 times, then switch to the opposite side.

Crunch with Leg Lifts

Purpose: To strengthen the lower abdominal muscles.

- Lie on your back with your knees bent.
- Place your left hand behind your head.
- Lift your head and left shoulder off the floor toward your right knee while lifting your right leg toward your chest.

Hold for 3 seconds, then return to the starting position. Repeat 10 times, then switch to the opposite arm and knee.

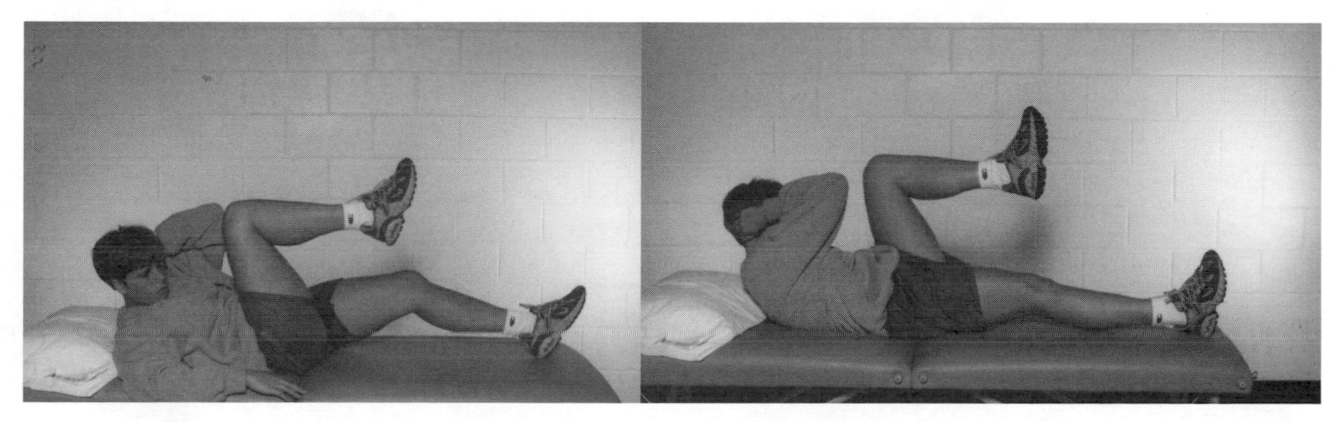

Crunch with Legs Off the Floor

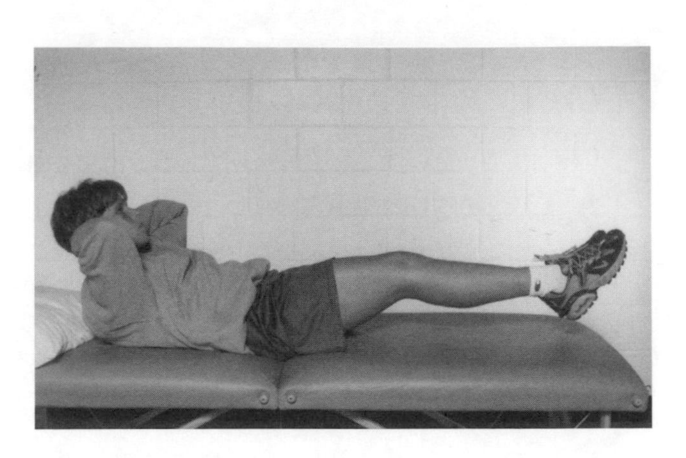

- Lying flat on your back, clasp your hands behind your head and lift your legs approximately 6 inches off the floor.
- Slowly raise your head and shoulders off the floor while keeping your lower and middle back flat against the floor. Try to get the entire shoulder blade to clear the floor.

Hold for 3 seconds, then return to the starting position

Note: This is a highly advanced exercise and should not be attempted until the previous abdominal exercise can be done for at least 30 repetitions of each.

Lower Back Strengthening

The following exercises progress from level 1 to 4. Level 1 is easiest. As you get comfortable with it, replace it with level 2, then 3, then 4.

Alternating Leg Lifts

Purpose: To strengthen the muscles of the lower back.

Level 1

- Lie face down on a firm surface.
- Lift your right leg up with your leg straight.

Hold leg in the upright position for 3 seconds and repeat 10 times. Switch legs.

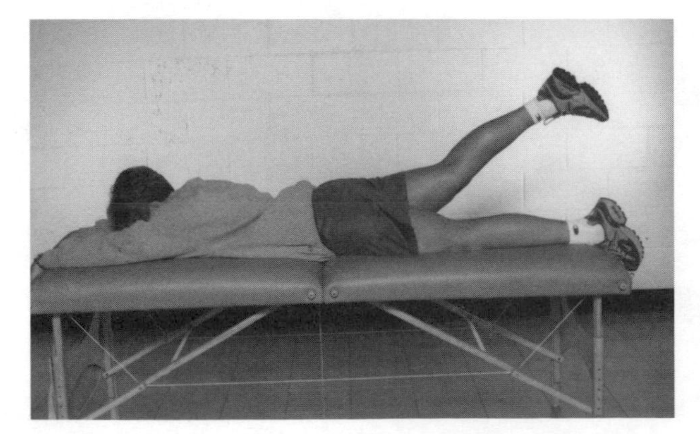

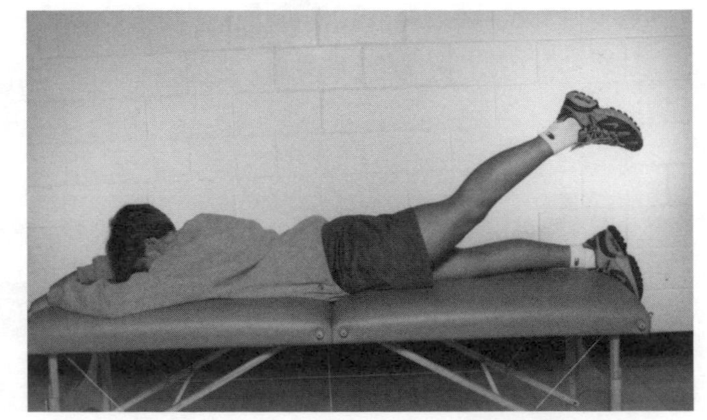

Alternating Leg and Arm Lifts

Level 2

- Place a pillow under your stomach. Lift your right arm and left leg toward the ceiling.
- Squeeze your buttocks as you lift your leg.

Hold for 3 seconds and repeat 10 times. Do the same with the left arm and the right leg.

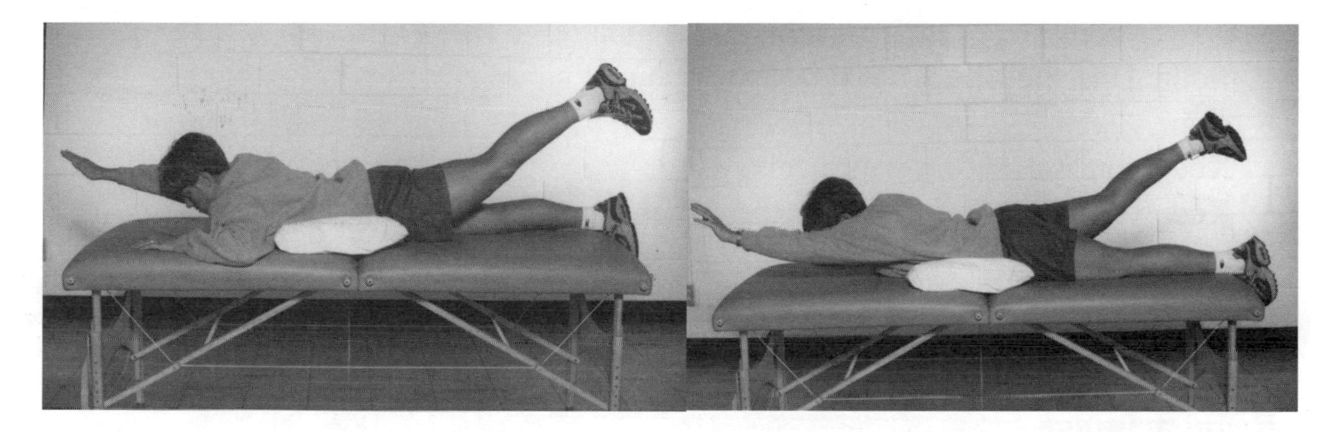

Alternating Leg and Arm Lifts on all Fours.

Level 3

- Start with both hands and knees on the table.
- Raise your right arm in front of you and your left leg straight behind you.

Hold for 3 seconds and repeat 10 times. Do the same with the left arm and the right leg.

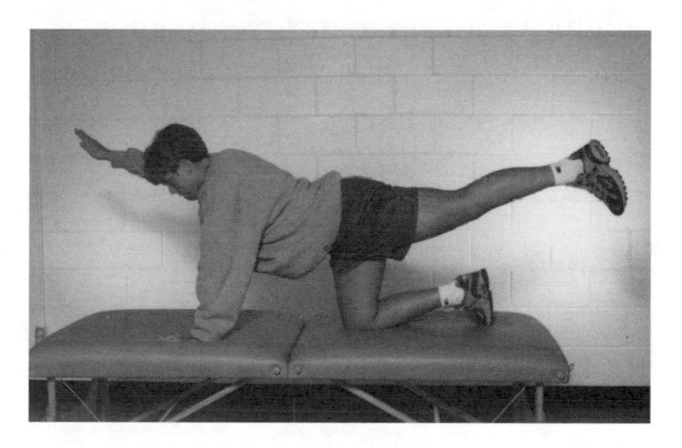

Back Hyperextensions

Level 4

- Lie on your stomach with your hands behind your head.
- Lift your head and chest off the floor by contracting your lower back muscles.
- Do not lift your waist or legs off the ground.

Hold for 3 seconds and repeat 10 times.

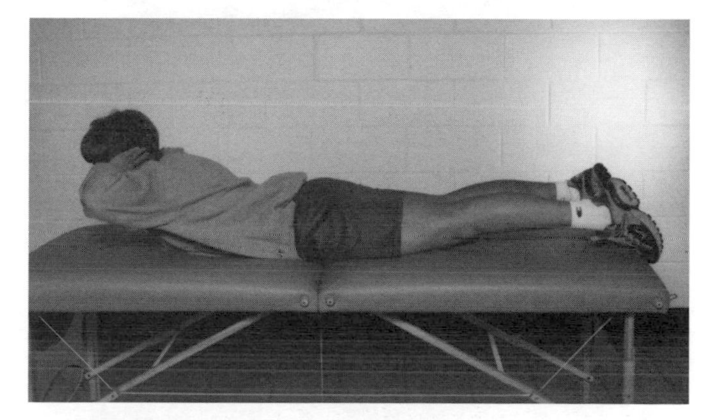

Wall Squats

Purpose: To strengthen the thigh muscles (front and back) and improve balance and coordination.

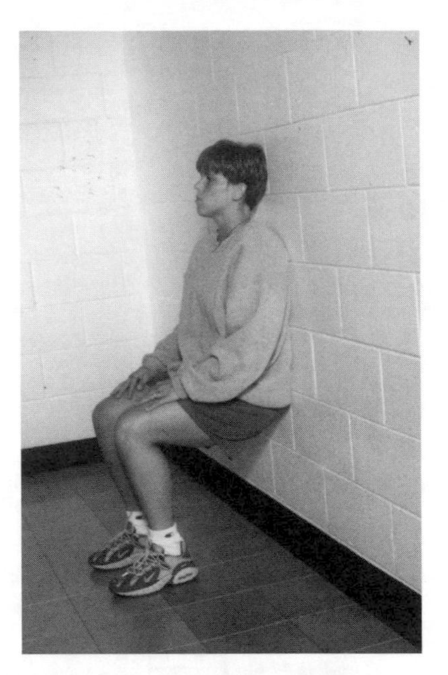

- Lean back against a wall and keep your feet at least shoulder width apart.
- Keep your heels on the floor and look forward.
- Bend both knees while your back maintains contact with the wall.
- Lower your body until your thighs are parallel to the floor. This should feel as if you are about to sit on a chair.
- Keep your weight on your heels.
- Keep your knees behind your toes when squatting down.

Hold for 10 seconds in the sitting position. Repeat 5 - 10 times.

Regular Lunge

Purpose: To strengthen the thigh muscles and improve coordination and balance.

- While standing, place your feet 6 to 12 inches apart and rest your hands on top of your right knee.
- Step forward with your right leg and bend your left knee towards the floor.

Hold for 1 second, then return to the standing upright position. Repeat 10 times.

Switch to the left leg and perform the same exercise.

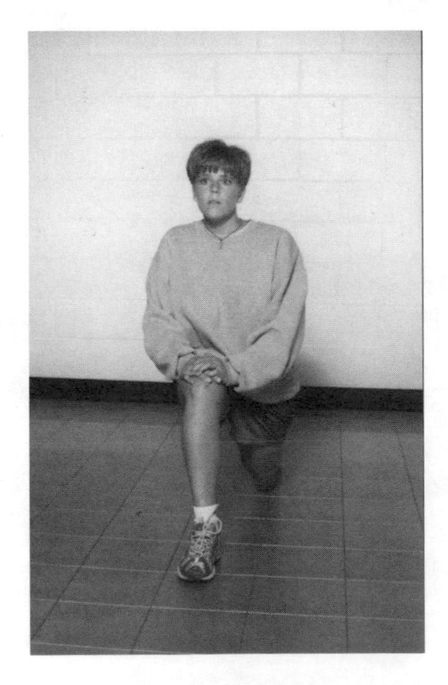

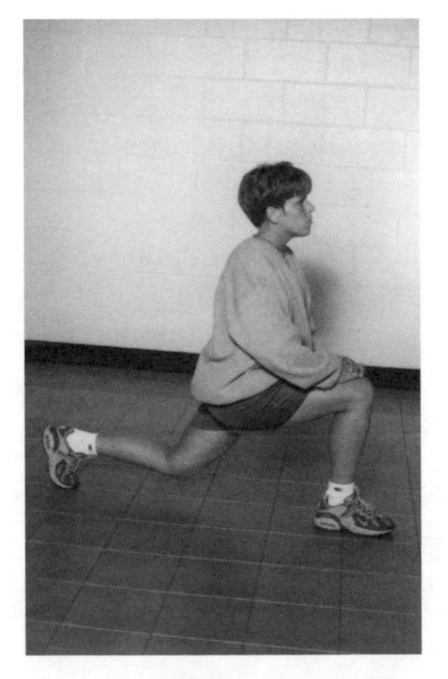

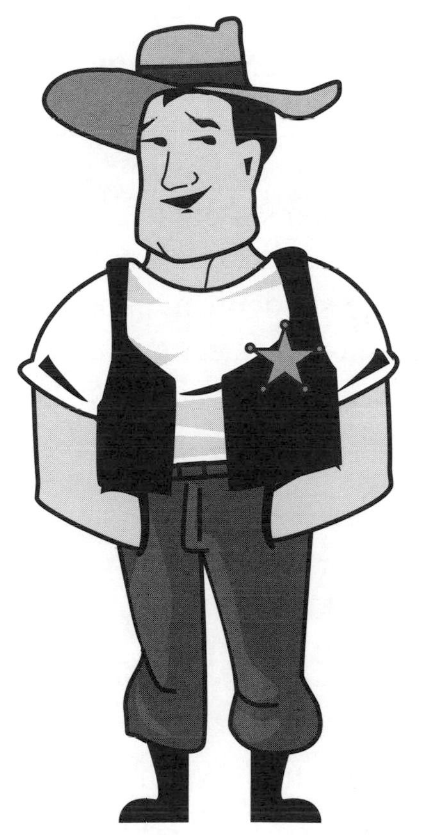

Sergio's Tip: Performing one exercise an hour during your workday will dramatically improve the health of your back.

Chapter 6

Posture: More Than "Sit up Straight"

Since Muskull felt so much better, he was anxious to hear what Sergio had to say.

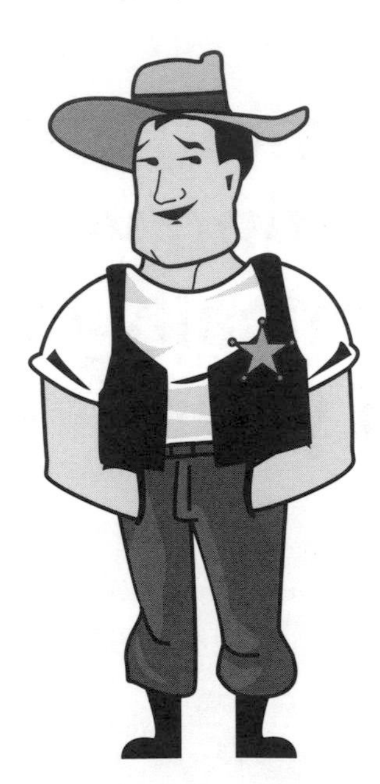

Sergio: There are several reasons why so many people are affected by disabling back pain. The most basic and overwhelming reasons for back injuries are postural problems. People often wonder, "How can posture cause a problem when I didn't have pain for all these years and now all of the sudden I'm in pain?" The answer is microtrauma. Microtrauma is the accumulation of small stressors that eventually wear down your lower back. These stressors might not cause lower back pain right away, but over time can eventually lead to a lower back injury.

Muskull: I feel funny and look kind of funny when I maintain a good posture!

Sergio: Most people perform their daily activities with poor posture. When attempting to sit or stand with proper posture they often feel awkward. Proper postural positioning may feel weird at first, but it is vital to maintaining a healthy body. If you make it a priority in your life, good posture will eventually feel natural.

Sitting Posture

Muskull: It feels natural when I slouch in my chair.

Sergio: Sitting slouched for long periods of time causes one of the worst stresses on your lower back. It places your spine in a flexed position, which forces disc fluid to the back of your disc. This consistent pressure placed on the disc fluid over time can lead to a bulging or herniated disc. Sitting slouched also stretches the ligaments of the back. Normally, the ligaments assist the muscles in protecting the spine from injuries. If the ligaments are overstretched, they will not support the back properly. This will lead to an earlier onset of back injuries.

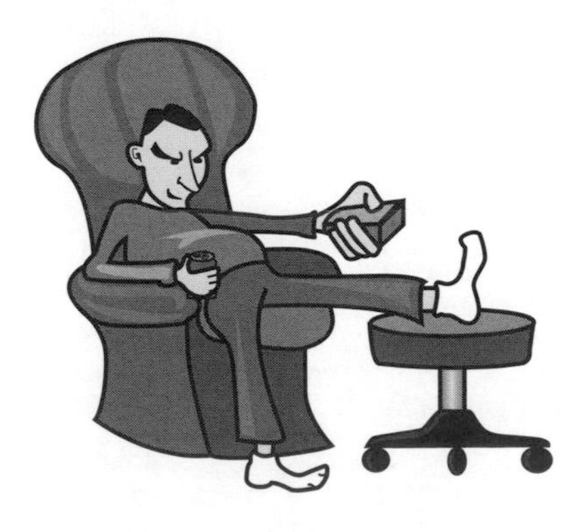

Sustaining Good Posture

Muskull: I started sitting up straight but after a while my back started to hurt again. Why did this happen?

Sergio: Good posture, although important, can be painful if you keep it the same throughout the day. Your postural muscles allow you to stay upright for long periods of time. However, if your posture is not adjusted several times a day, these muscles will fatigue. You can change your postural positioning ever so slightly to allow different postural muscles to work. There are several easy ways to adjust your posture. You can begin by adjusting the height of your chair or work surface or placing one foot on a stool when standing for long periods of time. Remember to alternate your feet. Changing your position every 30 to 60 minutes is fine. Just alternating between two favorite positions is enough.

Sergio's Tip: Perform one standing backbend every time you get up from sitting.

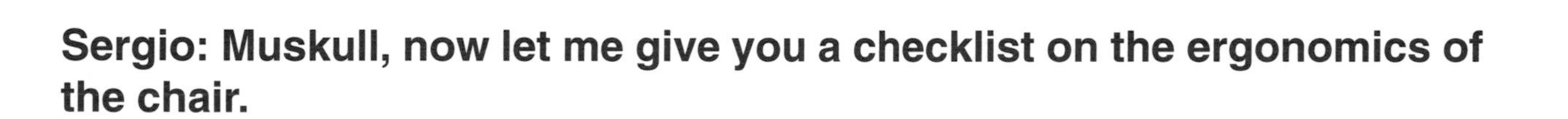

Sergio: Muskull, now let me give you a checklist on the ergonomics of the chair.

Muskull: What does the word ergonomics mean?

Sergio: Ergonomics is how you interact with your work environment. How you sit, stand, type, lift, etc. A work environment that is set up ergonomically correct will put less stress on the worker.

Ergonomics of the chair

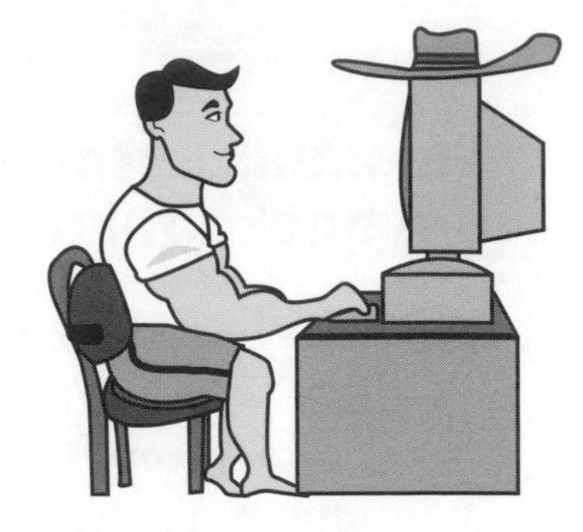

Sergio recommends that chairs or seating should:

1. Have the ability to adjust the height of the seat, armrests, and the position of the back.

   Rationale: To accommodate the shape and height of one's body.

2. Allow for the worker to rest his or her feet comfortably on the floor. If a person's workstation does not allow for this, then a footrest should be placed under the feet.

   Rationale: To take stress off the lower legs and back.

3. Have swivel seats to ease the ability to turn and reach for objects.

   Rationale: To reduce excessive reaching and twisting of the lower back.

4. Have good lower back support.

   Rationale: To help maintain the natural curve of the lower back and to encourage a more upright head and neck posture.

5. Have a seat pan (what you are sitting on) that is tilted slightly forward. The back of the chair should be on a slight angle higher than the front of the chair.

   Rationale: To help the lower back maintain its natural curve.

6. Have a seat pan that is not too long.

   Rationale: This may cause the worker's calf muscles to come in contact with the front edge of the seat pan. To avoid this, the worker might adopt a slouched sitting posture.

7. Have a lower back roll attached directly behind the lower back curve.

   Rationale: To support and maintain the lower back curve.

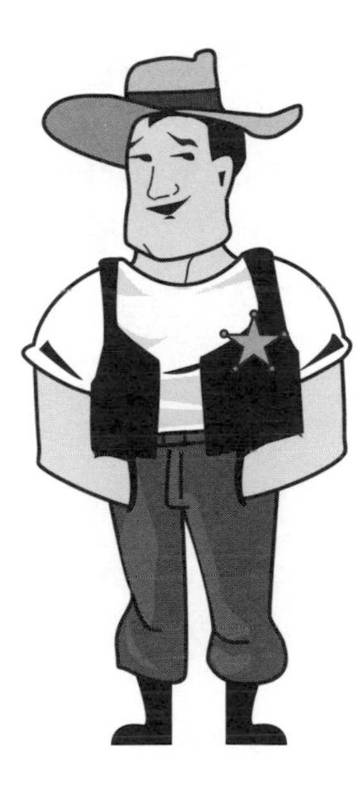

Sergio's Tip: You must sit in the chair properly. Sit up nice and tall. If you feel that you're starting to slouch, you should get up and take a stretch break.

Muskull: After slouching during sitting for so many years, why does my back hurt now?

Sergio: This is why your back hurts when you slouch: You're a creeper!

I don't mean to insult you Muskull. Creep is what occurs when the ligaments of the back are stretched too much. If you stretch a ligament for any period of time, it lengthens and eventually develops small tears. Over time, these ligaments become weak and are unable to support your spine, especially when sitting.

This is what creeping feels like:

You will feel an ache in the lower back.

This is how you get rid of creep:

Let the ligaments relax. Use the two exercises below to stop your ligaments from creeping.

Sit in a chair relaxed and slouched. Now sit as tall as you can and place your hand in the small curve of your back (refer to page 36).

Try to slouch with your arm behind your back. It should now be harder to slouch than when your arm isn't there. In place of your arm, you can place a lumbar roll (a lumbar roll helps maintain the natural curve in your lower back when you are sitting) on the back of the chair or you can roll up a towel and use it as a temporary roll.

Try to slouch with the rolled up towel or lumbar roll on the back of your chair. If it is more difficult to slouch, than the towel or roll is of good thickness and is supporting your back. If it is uncomfortable to sit with, it may either be too thick or not thick enough. Try adjusting the thickness.

At first, keeping the towel or roll in the small of your back for a whole day may be uncomfortable. Start by placing the towel or roll there for 15 minutes at a time and gradually increase the time of using the towel or roll until you are comfortable using it for an hour. This may take several days.

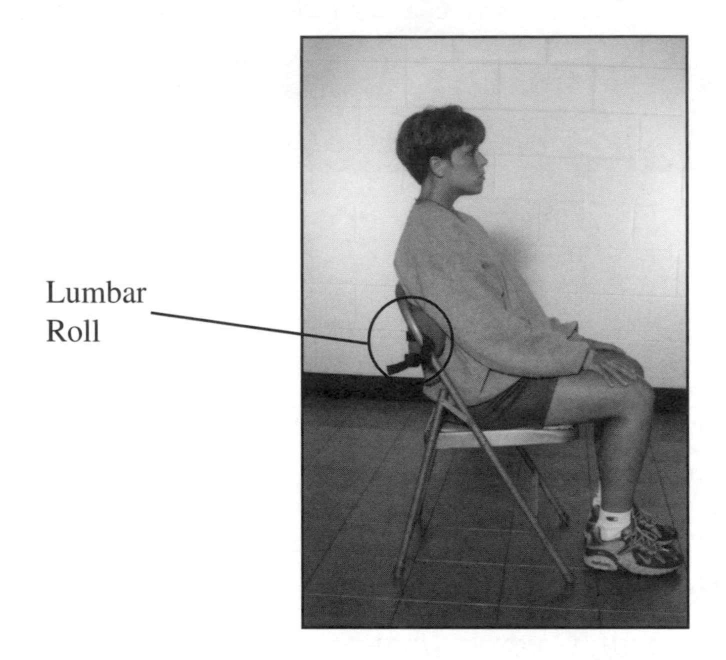

After sitting for an hour, you should stand up and do a standing back bend exercise.

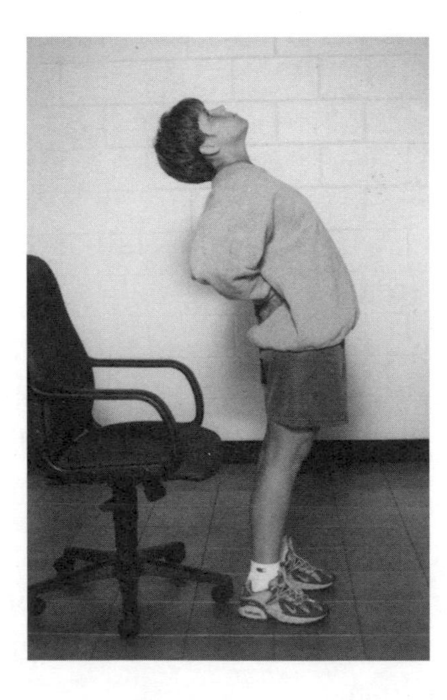

Muskull: Why does my back and leg hurt when I drive?

Sergio: When I used to have back problems, my back would ache while driving. On long drives, my thigh and leg would also hurt. When I would try to get out of the car, my back would sometimes stiffen up, and it would take me a while to straighten up. Once I started moving around, my leg and back would feel better. I could then continue my driving, but everything would eventually revert back and repeat itself. Sometimes, I would feel tingling, pins and needles or numbness in my legs.

Typically, when you drive, your back is in a slouched or bent position. This puts stress on the disc, ligaments and nerves. When they are stressed for too long, these structures begin to ache or tingle. This is a serious warning sign that they are stressed. You need to take the stress off the back.

This is what you can do about it. In most cars, you can adjust the seat to get closer or further from the steering wheel. In some cars, you can adjust the angle of the seat. But no matter how much you can adjust your position, it still may not be perfect. There are simple add-ons that you can use to make the car seat support your back. For one thing, using a lumbar roll for part of the car trip may help. The lumbar roll will support your back and keep you from slouching. On long trips, stop every 60 - 90 minutes to stretch your back. Second, your seat should be far enough so that your chest is at least 12 inches from the steering wheel.

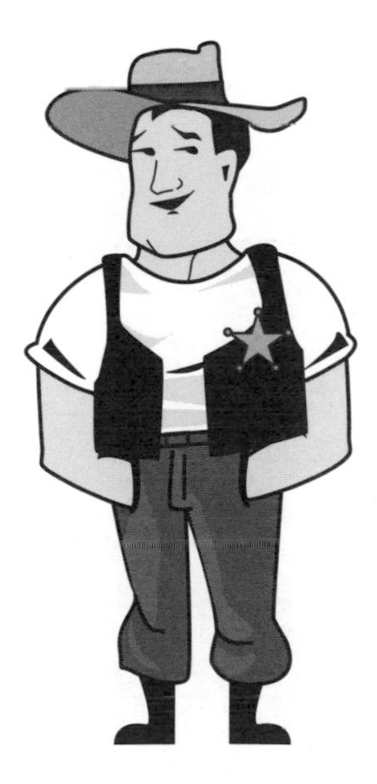

Sergio's Tip: Whenever you stop the car for gas or to run an errand, walk around the car and perform a standing backbend.

Standing Back Bends

Purpose: To take pressure off the back of your discs and relax the ligaments and muscles.

- Stand with your feet shoulder width apart.
- Place your hands on the middle of your lower back.
- Extend your back as far as your body allows you to, tilting your head back while keeping your knees straight.

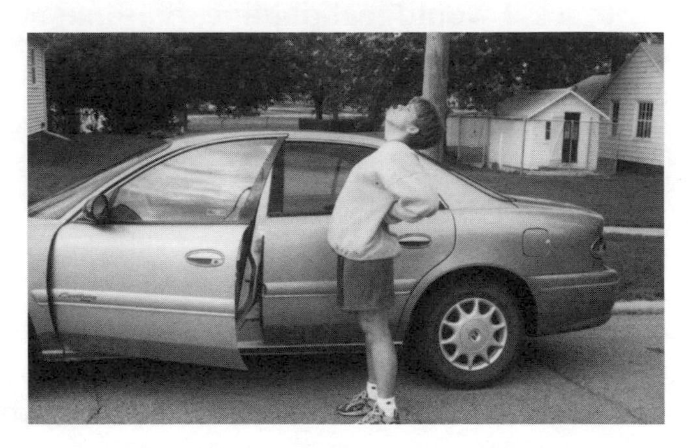

Hold for 1 second and repeat 5 times. This can be repeated many times during the day to counteract the forward bending postures.

Sergio's Driving Checklist

- Keep your chest at least 12 inches away from steering wheel.
- Position your knees so that they are higher than your hips.
- Keep the head rest up at the back of your head.
- Keep the lumbar roll at curve of the lower back.
- Keep the mirror raised up so that you have to straighten your neck to see it fully.
- Do not lower the mirror at the end of a work day. Rather, try to sit up taller to see from the mirror.

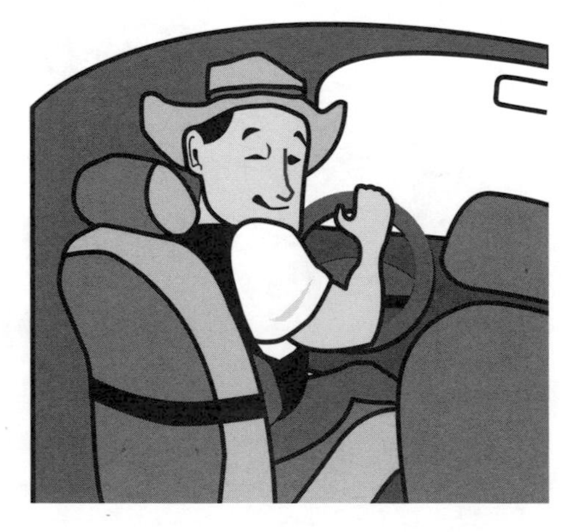

Sergio: You should also be aware of your posture when you stand for a long time.

Sergio's Standing Posture Checklist

1. When standing for a long period of time, place one foot on a stool or foot rest. Alternate feet periodically.

   Rationale: To decrease and alter the amount of stress placed on your lower back muscles.

2. When standing on a cement floor, wear shoes that provide good support and cushioning for your feet.

   Rationale: To reduce fatigue for your lower back muscles.

3. On cement floors place a floor mat where you are going to stand.

   Rationale: To reduce fatigue for your lower back muscles.

4. Try to stand an inch taller than you are used to.

   Rationale: To help you maintain a good posture.

5. Surfaces on which people stand for long periods should be designed to prevent slipping and should provide adequate traction and comfort.

   Rationale: To decrease the risk of falls.

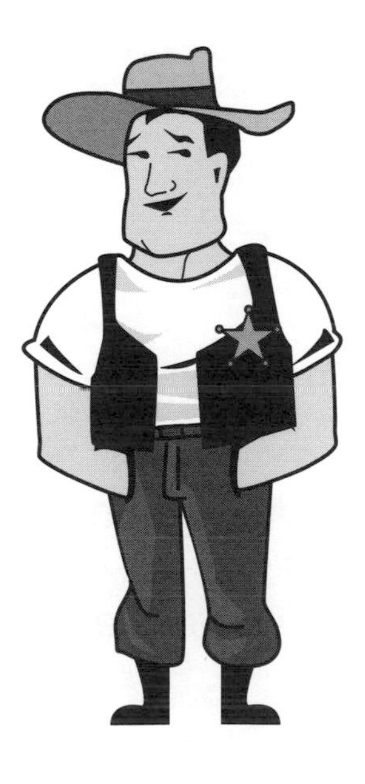

Sergio's Tip: Antifatigue floor mats, sit-stand stools and foot-rests can help make workers more comfortable at work.

Chapter 7

Lifting: More Than Just Bending Your Knees

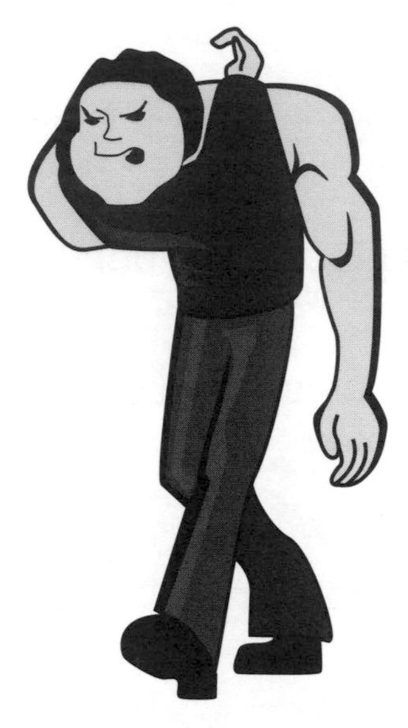

Muskull: Why did my lower back hurt when I bent forward to lift up a box and what should I do to prevent an injury the next time?

Sergio: Lifting improperly is one of the major causes of lower back pain. You can prevent back injuries by following my simple checklists when lifting.

Sergio's Lifting Checklist 1

1. Plan ahead. Know where you are going to place the object and clear that area and the path to that area before you lift.
2. Keep a wide base of support. Place feet shoulder width apart and one foot in front of the other. Place the object between both feet.
3. Bend your knees. Keep your back straight when lifting from the floor. Do not let your lower back bend forward.
4. Hold object close to your body.

Muskull: Does a lower back belt help during lifting?

Sergio: Not if you lift improperly! Lower back belts give a false sense of security for the person lifting. It will not help you if you do not lift properly. The proper use of a belt still requires good lifting technique. The belt allows you to tighten your stomach muscles to give additional support to the lower back.

Sergio's Lifting Checklist 2

1. Do not lift more than you can handle.

   Rationale: By lifting too much you place undo stress on your back and arms.

2. Give yourself enough recovery time in between lifts.

   Rationale: Without sufficient time between each lifting activity, your muscles will fatigue quicker, leaving you more susceptible to injury. There is no set period of time you should rest between lifts. Your best indication that it might be time to slow down is if your body starts to ache or if you feel fatigued.

3. Position item to be lifted in front of you to provide easy access.

   Rationale: It is less strenuous to lift something that is directly in front of you rather than off to the side.

4. Position item to be lifted between knee and shoulder height.

   Rationale: This is the best position to start. Items positioned on the ground and above shoulder height require more effort to lift.

5. Provide handles or cutouts to any box you are lifting.

   Rationale: This makes grasping and lifting easier.

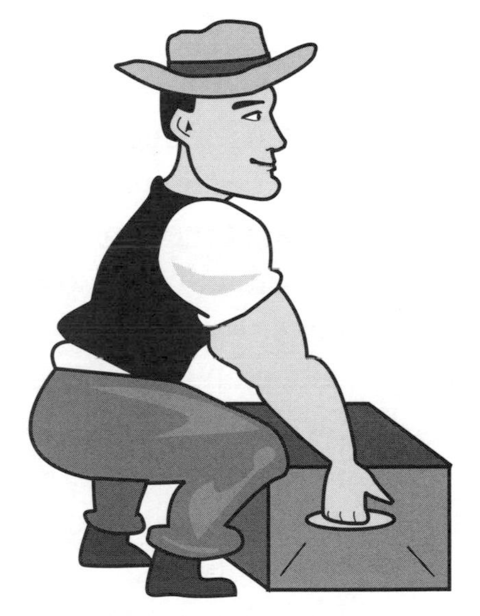

6. Carry item close to your body.

   Rationale: A 10 pound object places 100 pounds of stress on your lower back if you carry that object an arms length away from your body.

7. Decrease the distance or height the object needs to be moved.

   Rationale: The shorter the distance, the less energy needed.

8. Distribute weight within a box evenly.

   Rationale: This provides an even amount of stress to the muscles being worked.

9. Eliminate or minimize the amount of twisting that your body needs to do by taking the time to step and turn towards your target.

   Rationale: Lifting and twisting puts a lot of stress on the lower back muscles. If you can eliminate twisting, you will decrease the level of stress.

10. Use loaders, cranes and motorized material pallets when available to help move loads that are larger or heavier than one or two people can safely handle.

    Rationale: Many injuries occur when someone lifts more than they can handle.

11. Use hand carts or hand trucks.

    Rationale: Doing so decreases the likelihood for injury and the amount of energy spent moving and lifting the object.

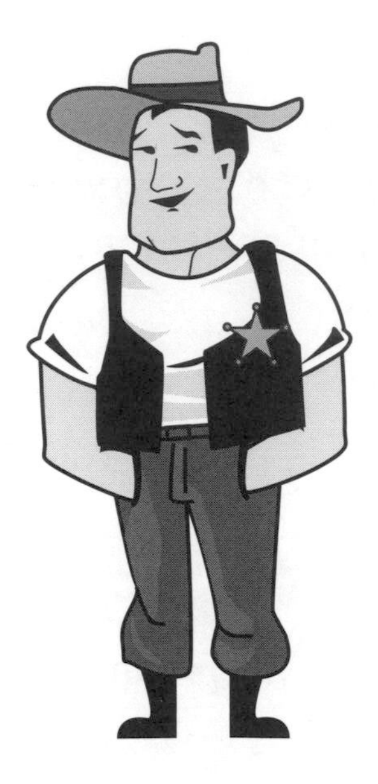

Sergio's Tip: Proper lifting will decrease muscle fatigue and reduce the likelihood for disc or muscle problems.

Golfer's Lift - This is a good lift to use when you need to pick up small and light objects with one hand.

- Face the object you are about to lift.
- Bend at the hip and knee, not at the waist, to maintain the normal curve of your lower back.
- Brace one free hand on your work surface or golf club to help stabilize your body.
- Allow your leg to extend back as you bend forward.
- Pick the object up, looking up as you straighten up.

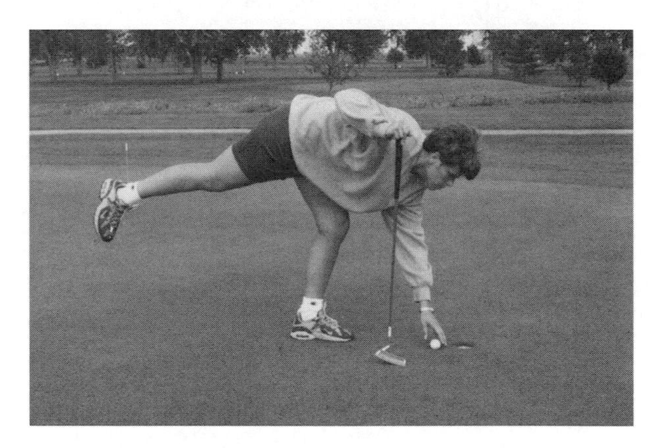

Pushing or Pulling Objects

It is generally easier to push than to pull an object. Regardless of whether you're pushing or pulling, use your legs, not your back, as leverage. Always seek help when pushing or pulling heavy objects.

Sergio: Improper lifting is a major cause of lower back pain. These are things to avoid:

- Do not bend at the waist. Bend at the knees instead.
- Do not keep your feet close together. This decreases your balance and strength.
- Do not carry objects away from your body. This places unnecessary stress on your spine.

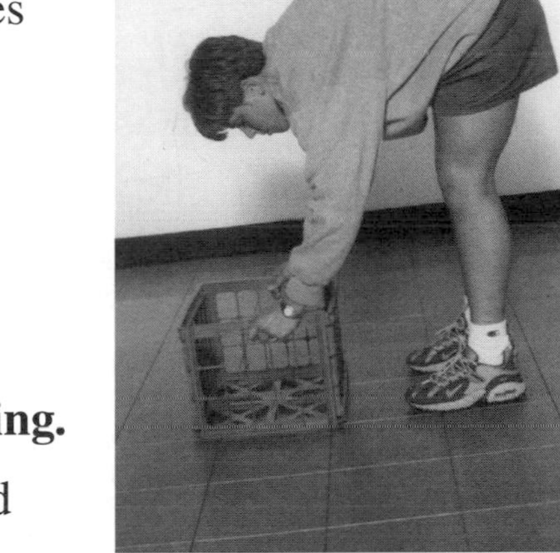
Improper Lifting

Sergio: This is why back injuries happen when lifting.

When bending and lifting, the muscles of the back and legs are used to support the body. If the object is too heavy, the muscles may over exert themselves and cause you pain. As you can imagine, straining to lift something heavy will cause a strain on your muscles. If your muscles are not prepared for the amount of work that has to be done, they will be injured. The muscle may tear or spasm from the heavy load. It is common to have muscle spasms in the back from too much or too heavy lifting. If the muscles fatigue or strain, they will not support the back and other injuries like sprains or disc injuries can result.

Sergio: This is what you should do when you initially feel pain.

After any initial injury, you should stop what you are doing. The most favorable and least stressful position for your lower back is the 90-90 position. The knees and hips are at 90 degree angles and are relaxed. Assume this position and place an ice pack on the part of the back that hurts. This should help speed up the healing process and decrease swelling to the area.

90-90 Position

Chapter 8

Ergonomics: Less Stress on Your Back.

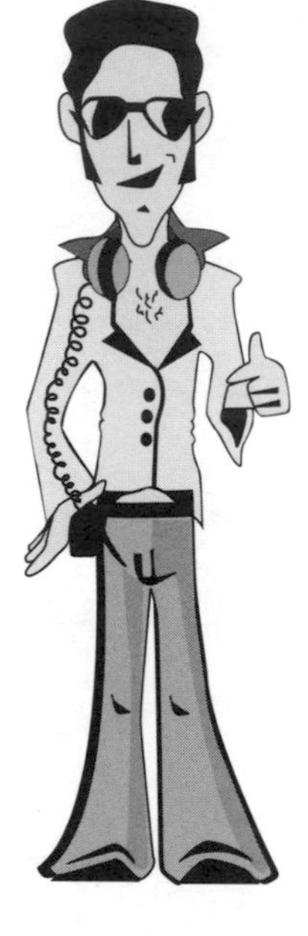

Disco: You know Sergio, my friend's office is designed completely different than ours.

Sergio: How is it different?

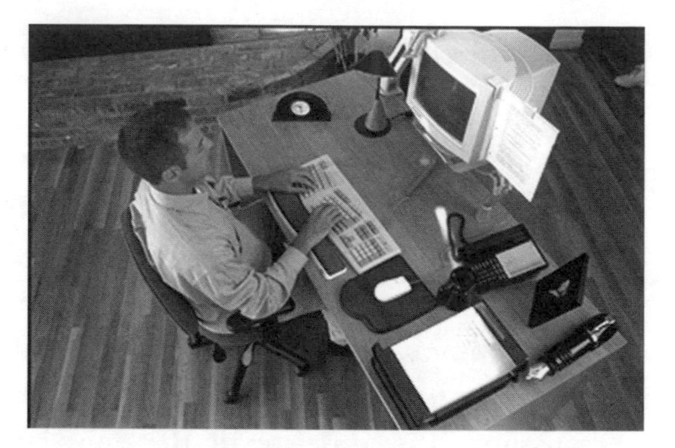

Disco: He told me his company just bought all new ergonomically designed computer workstations. They also gave each employee a copy of a book titled, "ErgAerobics:" Why Does Working @ My Computer Hurt So Much? which explains how to work ergonomically. What is ergonomics?

Sergio: Ergonomics refers to the way you set up and interact with your work environment.

Poor design of one's work environment can lead to increased fatigue, work stresses, and a greater likelihood of injuring oneself.

Good ergonomic design is simple know-how. Once you understand what part of your job causes you the most stress, try to rearrange your environment to minimize that stress. Buying the most expensive ergonomic equipment will not necessarily solve your problem. You must know how to use it and set it up properly to minimize work stress. Using the appropriate equipment and using it properly is the key to minimizing stress on the body.

Sergio's Ergonomic Advice for Your Lower Back

1. The work surface should be at your waist level. If its too low, raise it.
2. If a shelf is too high, use a step stool to reach an object on it. Constant reaching for objects will stress your shoulder tendons and back muscles.
3. Organize heavier loads on a shelf that is at waist level. Then load lighter objects on the upper and lower shelves.
4. When transferring materials, minimize the distance needed to travel and clear objects in your path.
5. If an object is too heavy, ask for help lifting it. If you find yourself arching your back backward when walking, it is a sure sign that you are probably lifting too much. Lighten the loads you need to lift if they are too heavy.

Work Habits

You can work in the most ergonomically correct work environment, but it will do you no good if you have poor work habits. Good work habits will minimize work stresses, decrease fatigue and improve productivity. The good work habits you achieve on the job must be carried out in your home environment as well.

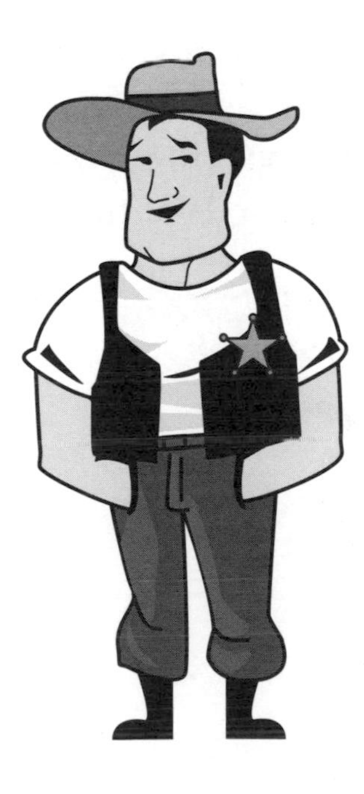

Sergio's Tip: By setting up your work environment properly you will lessen the stress on your body.

Sergio's Work Habits to Follow

1. Maintain a good sitting posture throughout the day.
2. Do not slouch. Change you're sitting posture ever so slightly every hour.
3. During prolonged periods of standing, alternate your feet on a footrest or stool.
4. Always use good body mechanics when lifting.
5. Always carry objects close to your body.
6. Do not twist your body to load an object.
7. Always step with your feet toward your object, never twist your back to turn.
8. Never lift an object that is too heavy. Ask for help if the object you are lifting is too heavy.
9. Perform one minute of stretching every hour.
10. Rotate different job tasks every hour to alternate work stresses placed on the body.
11. Never rush through a job. Take your time and do it right and safe.

Ergonomic Risk Factors and Corrective Recommendations for Your Lower Back

1. **RISK FACTOR: Sustained Sitting.** Sitting is one of the worst stresses for your lower back. Sustained sitting multiplies that stress. Sitting for prolonged periods of time can cause problems with your lower discs and postural muscles of your lower back.

   CORRECTIVE RECOMMENDATIONS: If you have to sit, try to find a comfortable chair with good lower back support. Also, get up from sitting one minute every hour and move around. If you do one standing backbend, you will reverse the stress placed on your lower back discs from sitting for long periods of time.

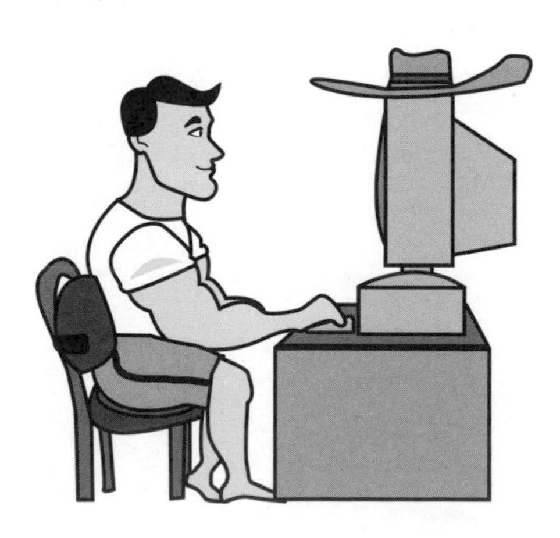

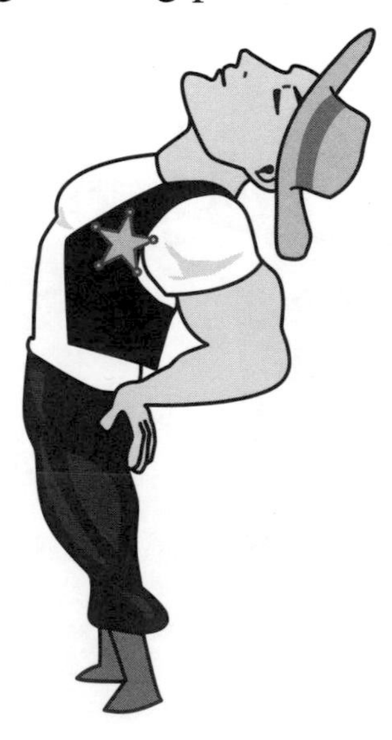

2. **RISK FACTOR: Sustained Standing.** Standing places stress on the postural muscles of your lower back. Sustained standing will cause these postural muscles to fatigue, potentially leading to an injury.

   CORRECTIVE RECOMMENDATIONS: Place a stool where you are standing and alternate your feet on this stool. This minimizes the stress placed on your lower back muscles. If no stool is available, place your foot up on what is available. Try not to stand greater than one hour at a time. Take a sitting break one minute of every hour or whenever you can.

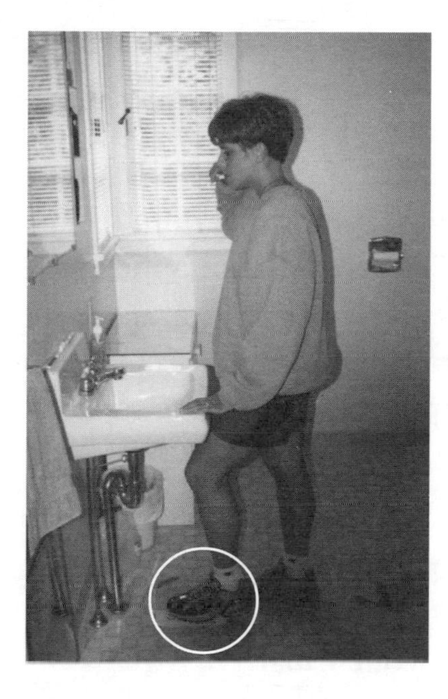

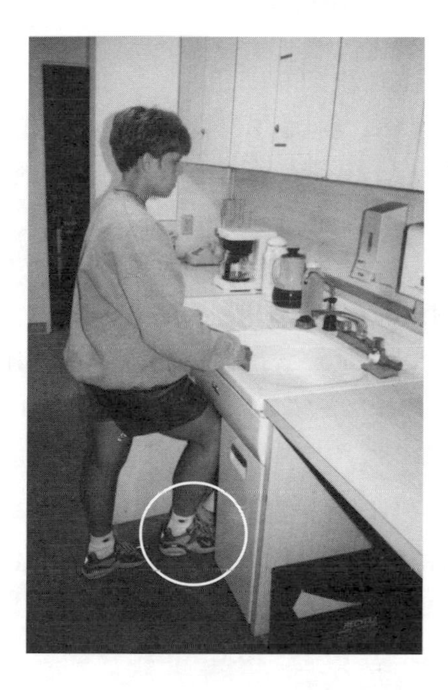

3. **RISK FACTOR: Poor Chair Design.** Sitting in a poorly designed chair puts significant stress on your lower back. It is more difficult to sit with good posture when sitting in a poorly designed chair.

   CORRECTIVE RECOMMENDATIONS: A good chair should have the following features: armrests, an adjustable seat, backrest and good lumbar (lower back) support. If you do not have a good ergonomically designed chair, add a lower back support (lumbar roll or towel) to the back of your chair.

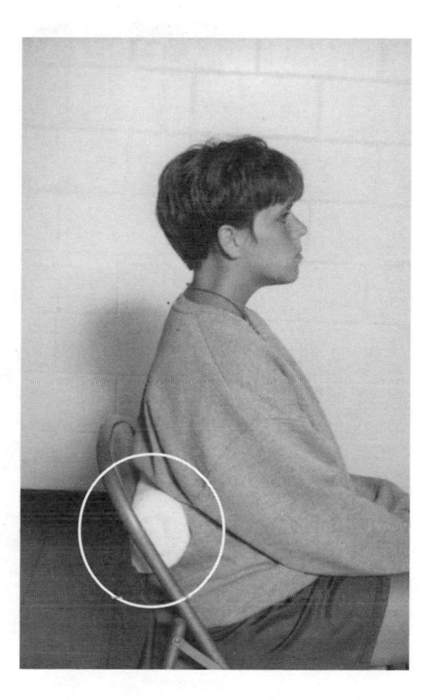

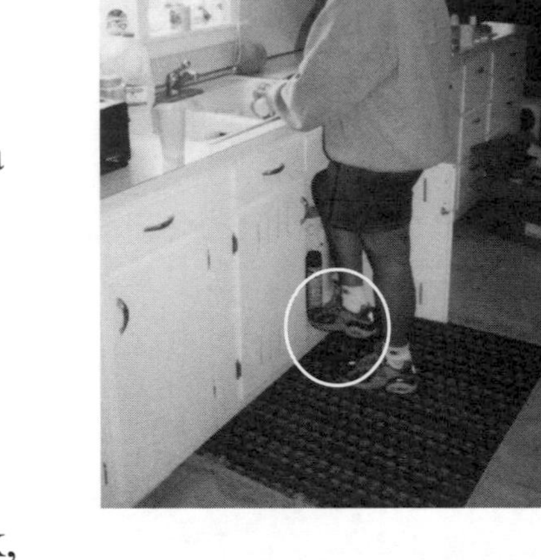

4. **RISK FACTOR: Cement Floors.** Standing on cement floors places greater stress on your legs and your lower back than standing on carpeted floors. Carpeted floors provide greater support and comfort for your feet. They also put less strain on your lower back and legs.

   CORRECTIVE RECOMMENDATIONS: If you have to work on cement floors make sure you wear a good shoe with good insole support. If a floor mat is available, use it at the spot where you need to stand throughout the day.

5. **RISK FACTOR: Forward Bending.** We bend forward most of the time. When we sit, wash at the sink, drive, eat, watch TV or pick up objects, we perform forward bending. It is a much more common activity than backward bending. This movement applies pressure on the front of the discs. The theory is that this pressure pushes the fluid to the back of the discs, which can cause the discs to lose their normal shape. When the discs change shape, they can press on a nerve. This repeated activity could also cause stress to lower back muscles.

   CORRECTIVE RECOMMENDATIONS: Try to arrange objects you are working with between your waist and shoulder to avoid forward bending. If your work surface is too low, raise it. If you are constantly lifting items, make sure you use good body mechanics. Bend at your knees not at your waist.

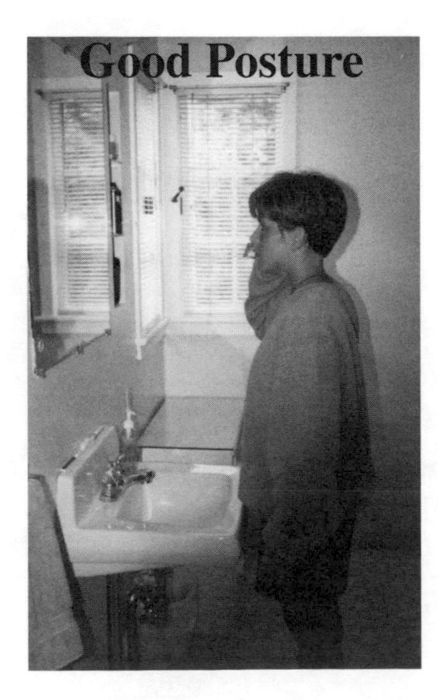
Good Posture

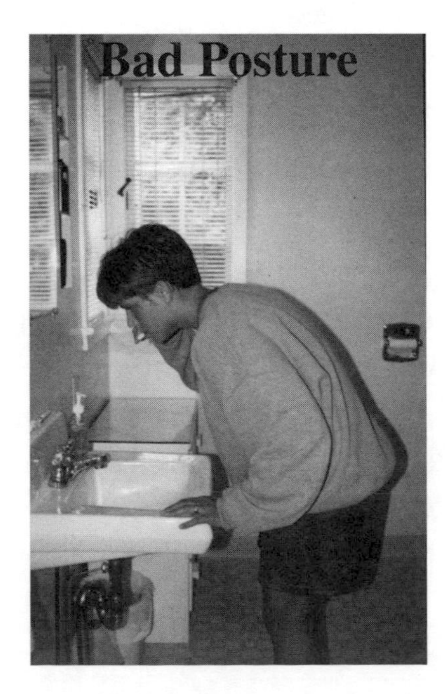
Bad Posture

6. **RISK FACTOR: Poor Sitting Posture.** Sitting slouched for long periods of time applies one of the worst stresses on your lower back. It places your spine in a flexed position, which forces disc fluid backward. This consistent pressure placed on disc fluid over time can lead to a bulging or herniated disc(see page 21).

   CORRECTIVE RECOMMENDATIONS: To reverse the stress placed on your discs during sitting, it is advisable to perform a standing backbend every time you stand up after sitting. This pushes the fluid from the back wall of the discs to a more central position. If you find yourself starting to slouch, stand up and move around. You should always try to sit up taller than normal.

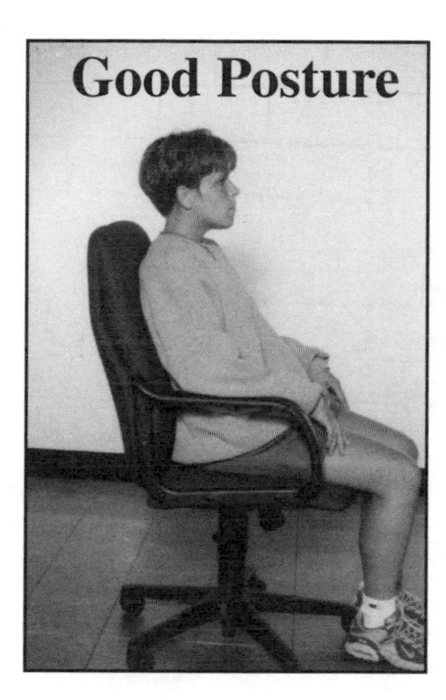

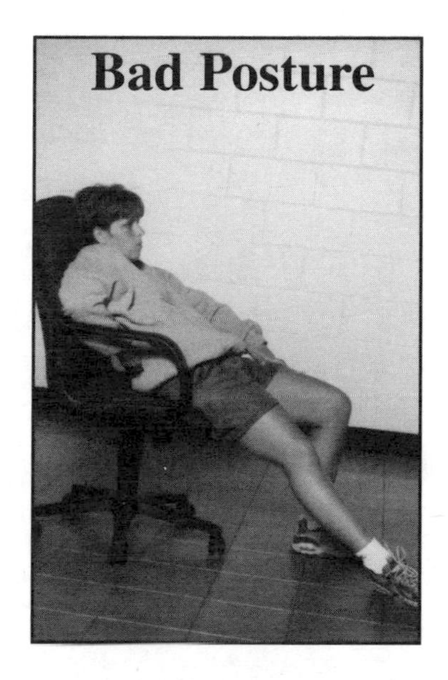

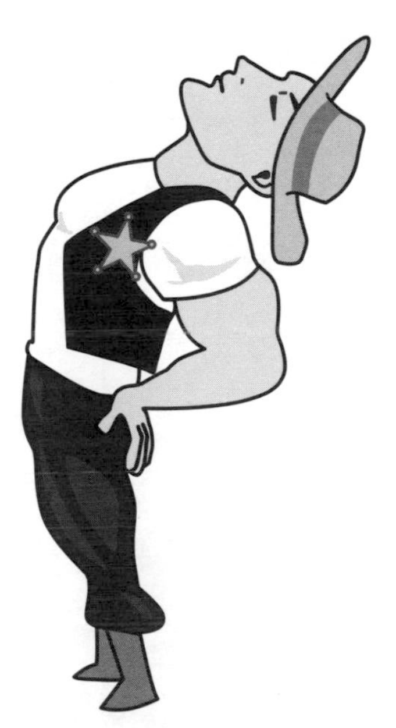

Sergio's Tip: Perform one standing backbend every time you stand up after sitting.

7. **RISK FACTOR: Twisting.** Turning your torso while keeping your legs stiff strains the back muscles and puts pressure on the joints of your lower back.

   CORRECTIVE RECOMMENDATIONS: It takes only about a half-second longer to step and turn rather than twist.

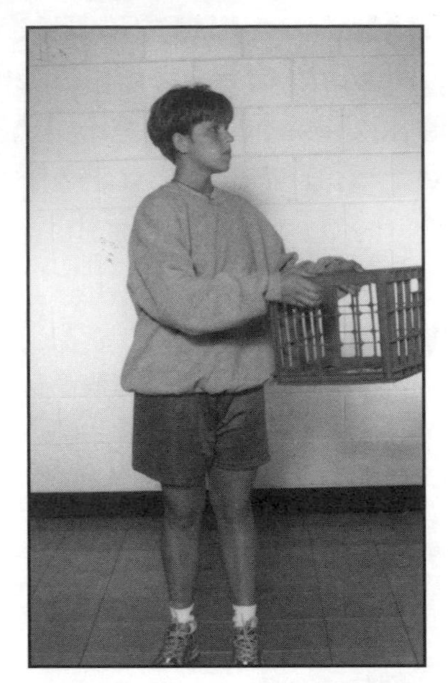

8. **RISK FACTOR: Lifting Excessive Loads.** This will place a lot of stress on the lower back muscles. Lifting loads you can not handle will cause the muscles to fatigue quicker. If you are arching your back when carrying an object, it probably is too heavy for you.

   CORRECTIVE RECOMMENDATIONS: Lighten the loads you lift. Initially, your productivity may decrease, but as time goes on it will increase. If there are any mechanical lifts available, use them to lift very heavy loads. If there is someone else around, ask him or her for help.

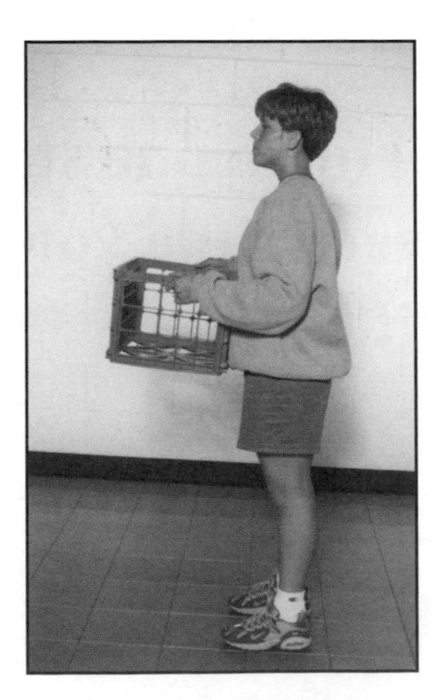

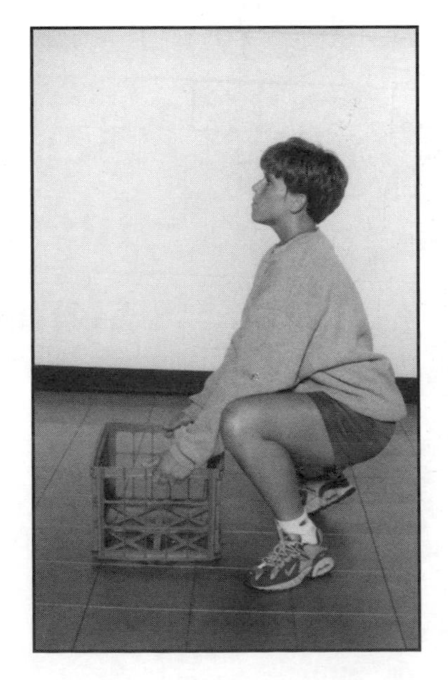

Chapter 9

Leisure Activities: Give Your Back a Break

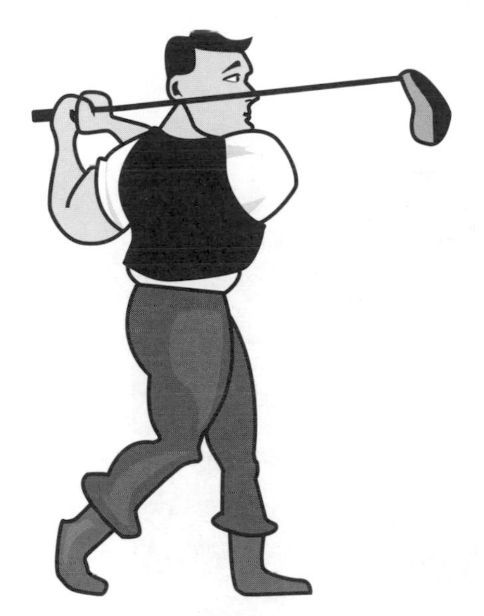

Golf Without Back Pain

Sergio: I love to play golf. Like many athletes, I did not associate physical injuries with golf. After all, contact sports like football and hockey seem to be more physically challenging, so injuries logically might occur more. But even though golf is not a contact sport, back injuries are the most frequent injury of golfers. The twisting and jerking movements in one direction only, can put a golfer in danger of serious back pain. Also, remember that throwing one's driver after shanking a ball into the woods can hurt one's back. Here is some helpful information on how to prevent lower back pain during and after you play golf:

Sergio: When you play golf you repeatedly bend forward at the waist. You bend forward when you putt, pick up your ball, carry the clubs on your back and lift your clubs out of your car. Even between golf swings when you sit in your golf cart, you place your spine in a forward bent position. Here is a checklist I follow to help maintain the health of my lower back while golfing.

Sergio's Golf Checklist

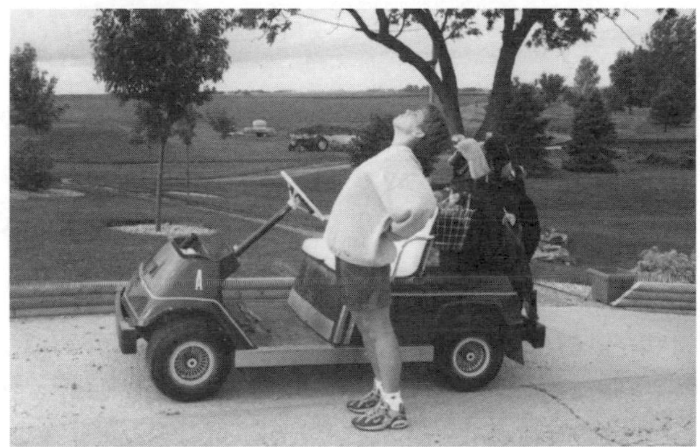

1. Every time you get out of your cart perform a standing backbend.

   Rationale: This will reverse the stress placed on your lower back from sitting in the cart.

2. When getting your clubs out of the trunk of your car, bend from your hips or on one knee. Do not bend with a rounded back.

   Rationale: This will minimize the stress on your lower back muscles during lifting.

3. Always carry the clubs near your body.

   Rationale: Let's estimate your golf clubs to weigh 15 pounds. If you carry your clubs close to your body, they place 15 pounds of stress on your back. If you carry those same clubs an arms length away from your body, you will place 10 times (150 pounds) the amount of stress on your back.

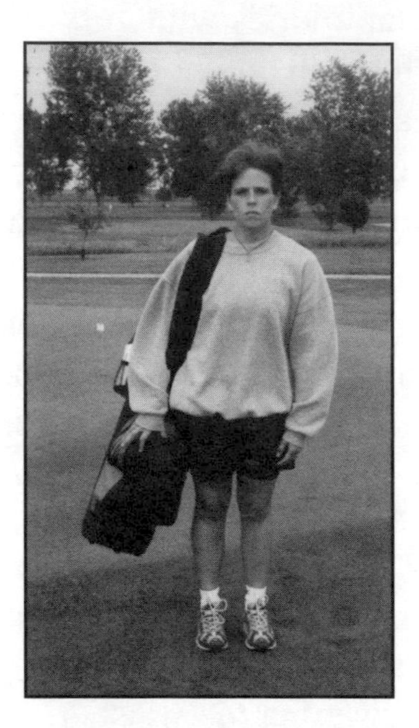
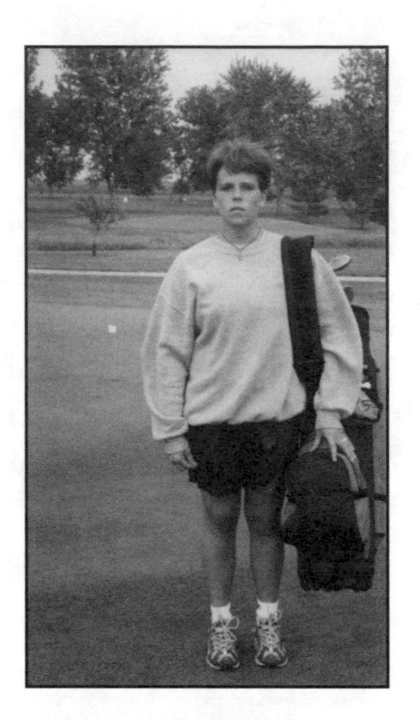

4. Use the back strap and carry your golf clubs over both shoulders. If you do not have a back strap, periodically alternate shoulders while you carry the golf clubs.

   Rationale: Back straps evenly distribute the weight of your bag across your back. This minimizes the chance of a muscle injury.

5. When picking up your golf clubs from the ground, remember to bend your knees. Keep your back straight at all times with only a slight arch in your lower back.

   Rationale: Lifting properly greatly decreases the likelihood of a lower back muscle strain.

6. Before playing golf, perform stretching exercises to loosen up your muscles, especially back muscles.

   Rationale: You will perform better with your muscles properly warmed up. You are also less likely to suffer a muscle pull.

7. After every couple of holes, or while waiting to putt or tee off, perform a couple of standing backbends.

   Rationale: This reverses the stress placed on your muscles and your lower back discs from repetitively bending forward during your golf game.

8. Do not bend over at your waist to pick up your ball. When picking up your ball,

either bend and squat at your knees or bend forward from the hip, keeping one leg straight (golfer's lift).

Rationale: Doing this places a minimal amount of stress on your lower back during lifting.

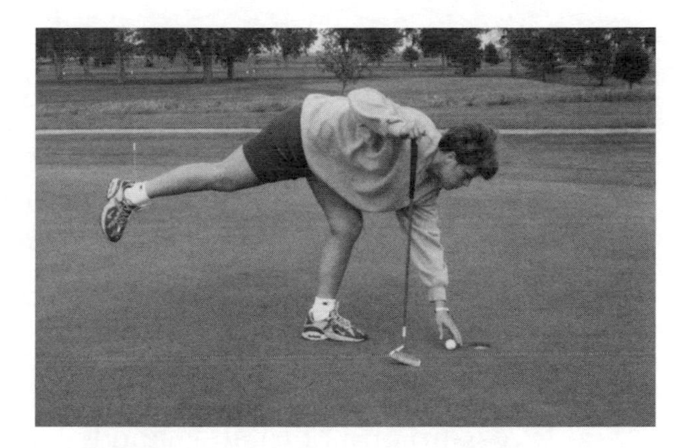

9. Limit riding in the golf cart. Walk briskly from hole to hole.

   Rationale: Reduces the risk of your muscles getting tight. Sitting reinforces the forward bending posture at the waist.

10. If you have to ride, use a lumbar roll and sit upright.

    Rationale: Using a lumber roll helps to reinforce good sitting posture.

11. When you finish playing, do not slump in your car or at home. Golfers are usually fatigued after a round of golf, making them vulnerable to back injuries even when they are relaxing. Maintain the same postural habits you had while playing golf.

    Rationale: Maintaining good posture in every thing you do is vital to preventing injury. Pretty soon doing your normal activities with proper posture and body mechanics will feel normal to you.

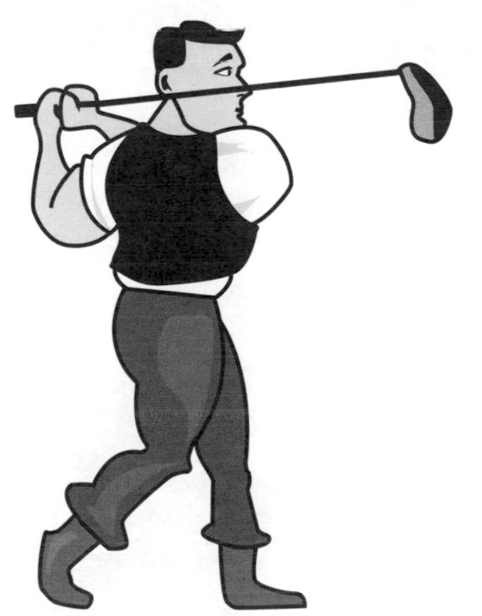

Sergio: Here are a couple of exercises to incorporate into your golf game.

Prone Press Ups

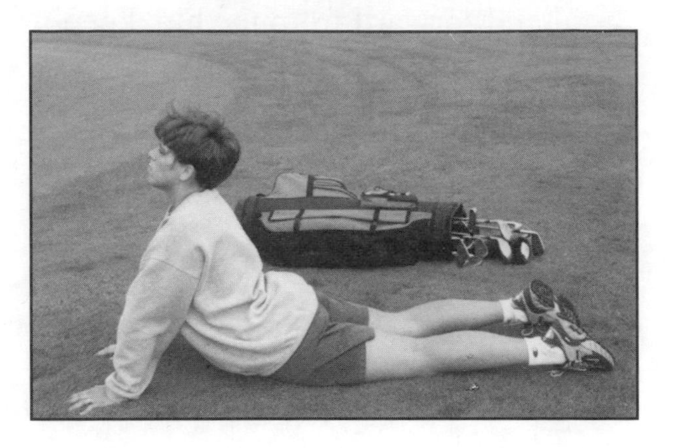

Purpose: To extend the lower back (counteract constant sitting). This exercise can be attempted if resting on your elbows is comfortable.

- Lie on the floor face down with your arms bent and hands flat on the floor by your shoulders.
- Press up on your hands and try to sustain your body weight on your arms while relaxing your hips and back muscles.

Hold for 1 second in extended position and repeat 5-10 times. This can be repeated many times during the day to counteract the forward bending postures.

Sitting Rotation Left

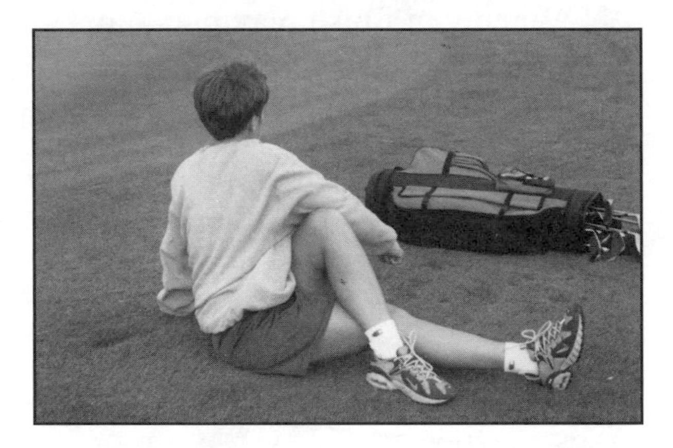

Purpose: To stretch the muscles on the right side of your lower back.

- With your right leg straight in front of you, bring your left leg over your right knee with your left knee bent.
- Turn your upper body to the left and place your right arm over your left knee.

Hold for 20 seconds at the end range position. If this stretch hurts, you are probably stretching a little bit too far.

Sitting Rotation Right

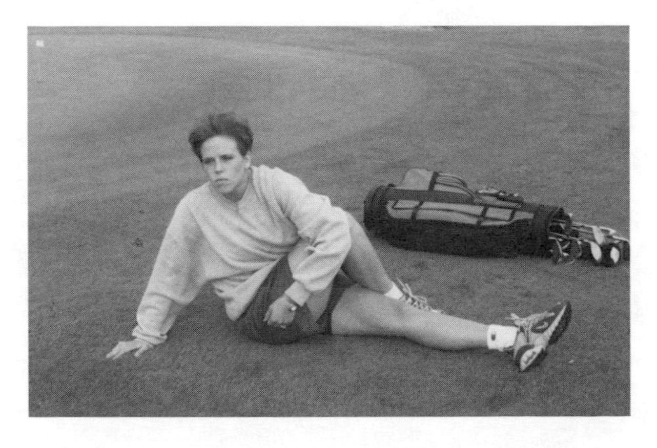

Purpose: To stretch the muscles on the left side of your lower back.

- With your left leg straight in front of you, bring your right leg over your left knee with your right knee bent.
- Turn your upper body to the right and place your left arm over your right knee.

Hold for 20 seconds at the end range position. If this stretch hurts, you are probably stretching a little bit too far.

Standing Back Bends

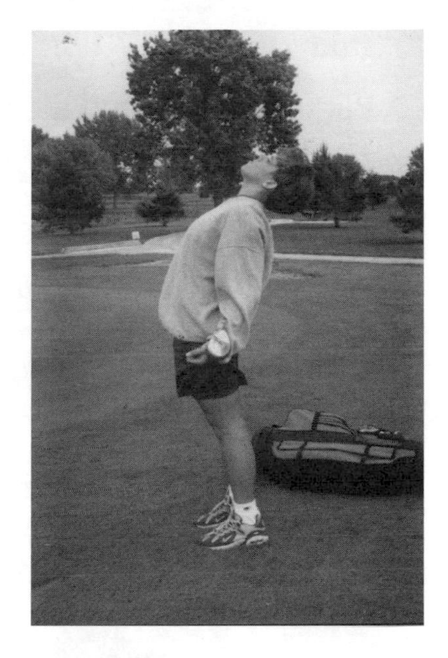

Purpose: To take pressure off the back of your discs and stretch the front ligaments and muscles.

- Stand with your feet shoulder width apart.
- Place your golf club straight across your lower back.
- Leading with your head, lean back as far as possible. Keep your knees straight during this exercise.

Hold for one second and repeat 10 times. This can be repeated many times during the day to counteract the forward bending postures.

Standing Side Bend Right & Left With Golf Club

Purpose: To stretch the muscles on the left and right side of your back.

- Hold a golf club straight across your lower back so that you feel the club gently touching your lower back.
- With each hand grab the end of the golf club.
- Bend over to the right side with the club on the right side of your body moving lower as the club on the left side of your body raises higher. Hold for 10 seconds at the end range position. Now stretch the opposite way.

Note: If this stretch hurts, you are probably stretching a little bit too far.

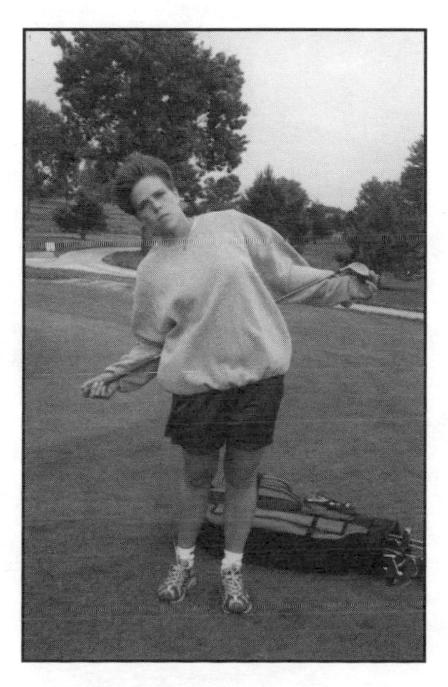

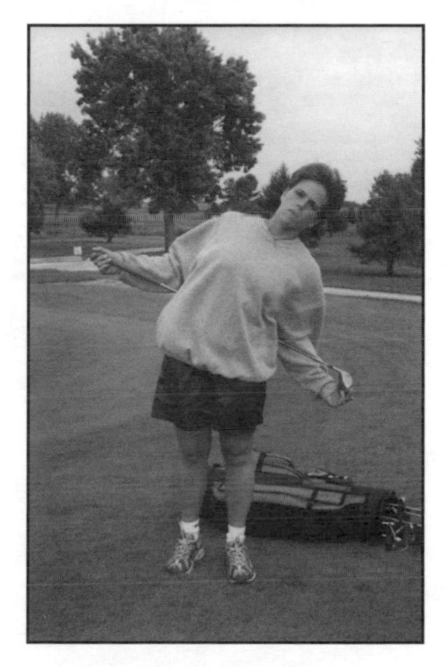

Body Rotation Right & Left With Golf Club

Purpose: To stretch the muscles on the left and right side of your lower back.

- Hold a golf club straight across the lower part of your back so that you feel the club gently across your lower back.
- Try not to move your legs. Only rotate your upper body and waist.
- Rotate your whole upper body toward the right, with your feet firmly planted and your knees straight.

Hold for 20 seconds at the end range position. Now stretch the opposite way.

Note: If this stretch hurts you are probably stretching a little bit too far.

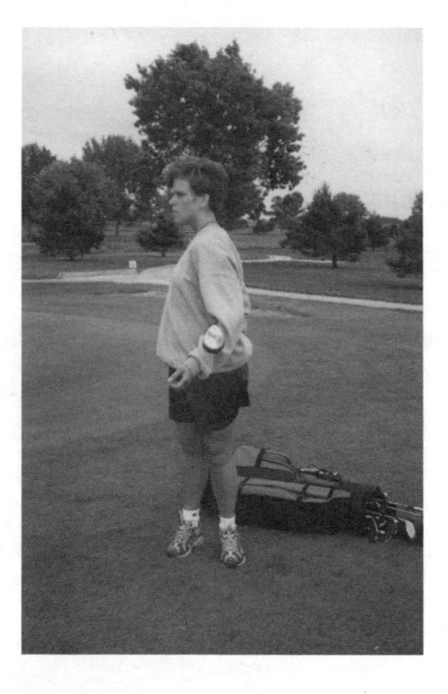

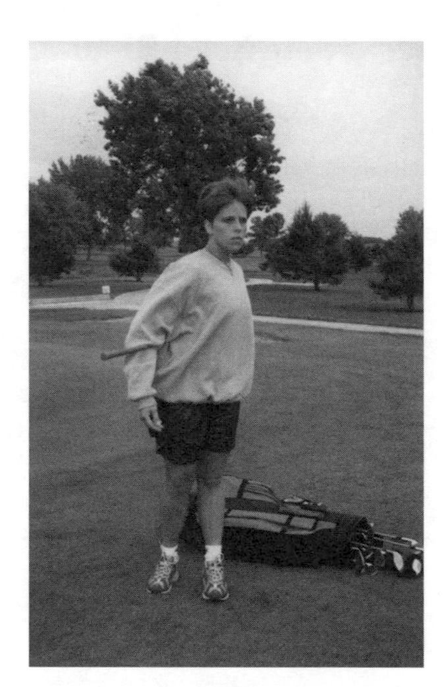

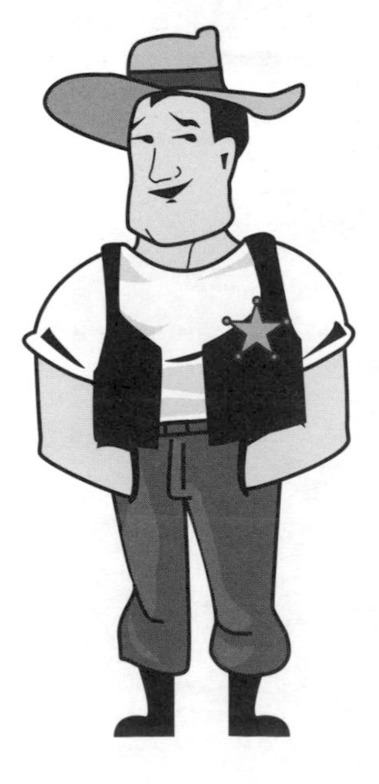

Sergio's Tip: Perform a standing backbend every time you get out of your golf cart.

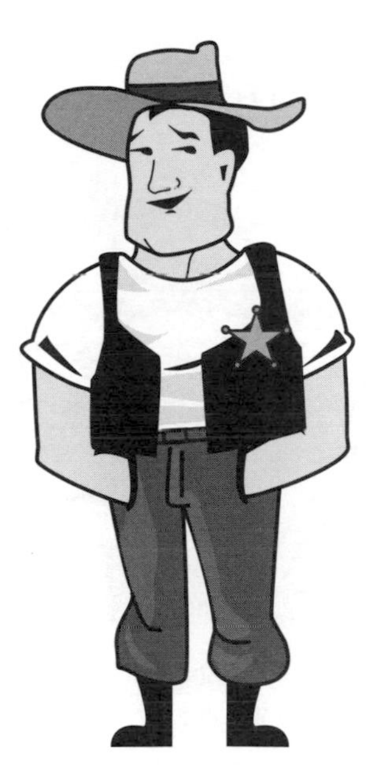

Gardening Without Back Pain

Sergio: I love to work on my garden and backyard. But, this seemingly harmless activity can actually contribute to chronic back pain.

Whether you're mowing your lawn, planting flowers, fertilizing or doing other jobs, gardening could put a lot of stress on your lower back. The problem lies in the position of your body. During yard work you need to repetitively bend forward and generally sustain this position for long periods of time. Here is a checklist I follow to help maintain the health of my lower back during gardening and yard work.

Sergio's Gardening and Yard Work Checklist

1. When working close to the ground, bend down on one knee. Do not bend forward at the waist.

   Rationale: Repetitive forward bending at the waist can cause a muscle pull or disc problems.

Good Body Mechanics

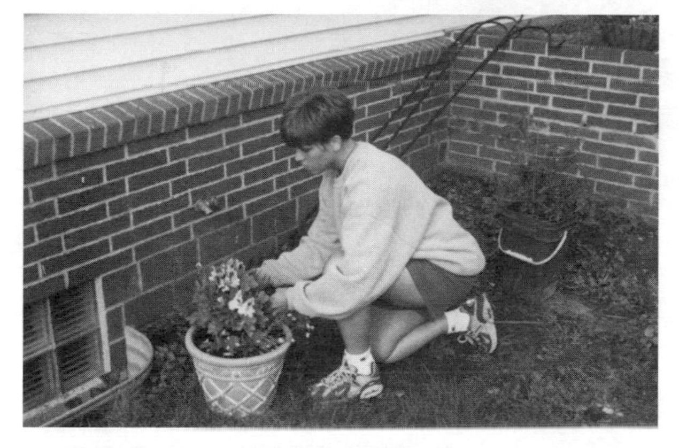

Bad Body Mechanics

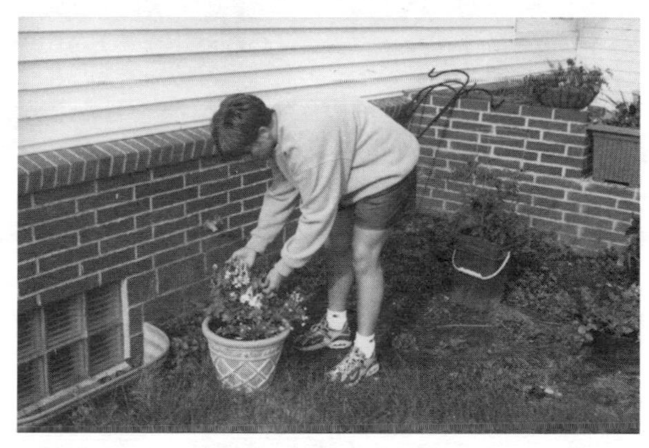

2. When picking a small item off the ground, keep one leg straight while bending forward from the hip (golfer's lift, page 60) or bend at your knees, not your waist.

   Rationale: Repetitive forward bending at the waist can cause a muscle strain or disc problems.

Good Body Mechanics | **Bad Body Mechanics**

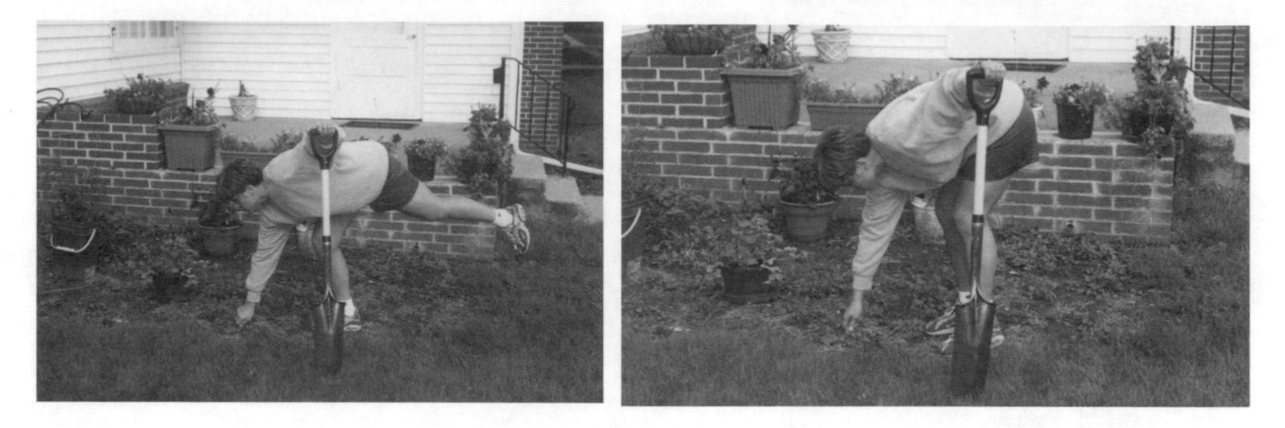

3. Periodically perform a standing backbend.

   Rationale: Doing so reverses the stress placed on your lower back and discs from repetitively bending forward.

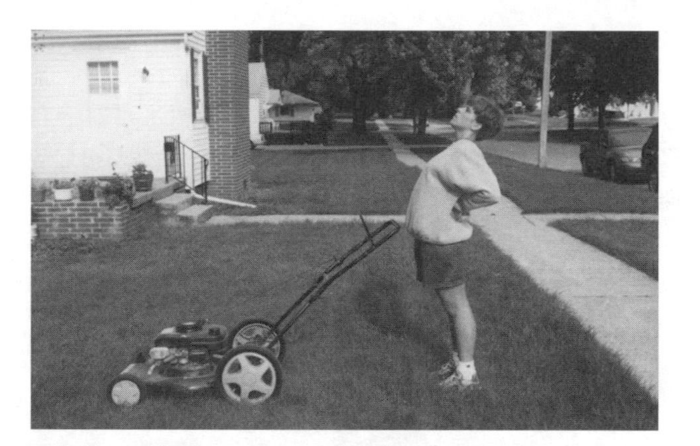

4. When mowing the lawn, keep your back straight.

   Rationale: Maintaining a good posture during work will minimize your chance for a lower back injury.

Good Body Mechanics | **Bad Body Mechanics**

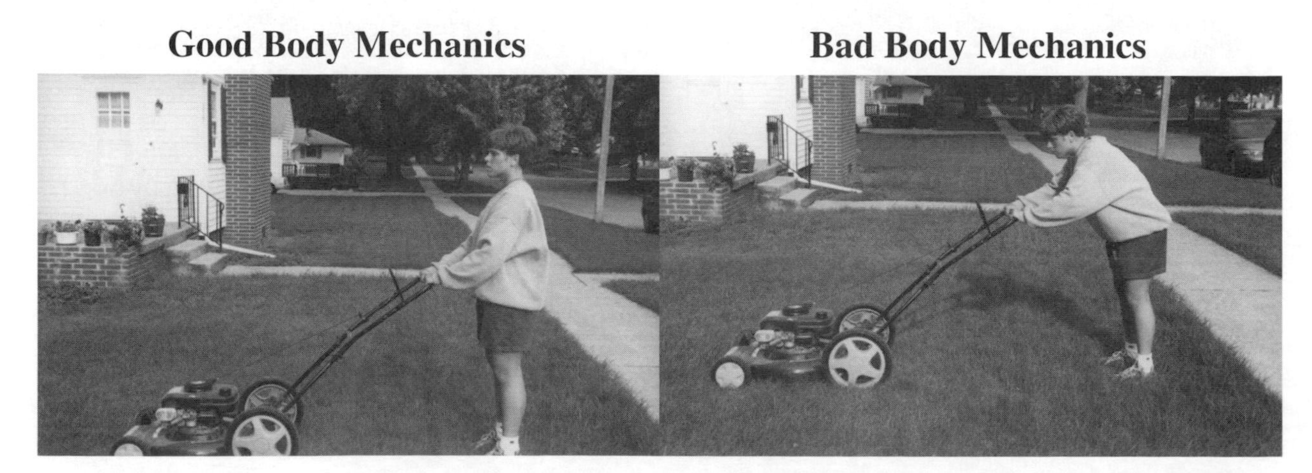

5. When carrying objects, keep what you are carrying close to your body.

   Rationale: If you carry an object that weighs 10 pounds an arms length from your body, you are placing about 100 pounds of stress on your lower back.

6. Pushing is easier on your lower back than pulling, so always try and position yourself to push rather than to pull.

   Rationale: The less energy needed to perform an activity, the less the muscles will fatigue.

7. Whenever cleaning difficult to reach objects, use a ladder or a step stool.

   Rationale: This places less stress on your shoulders, neck and upper back, therefore there is less stress on the lower back.

Good Body Mechanics

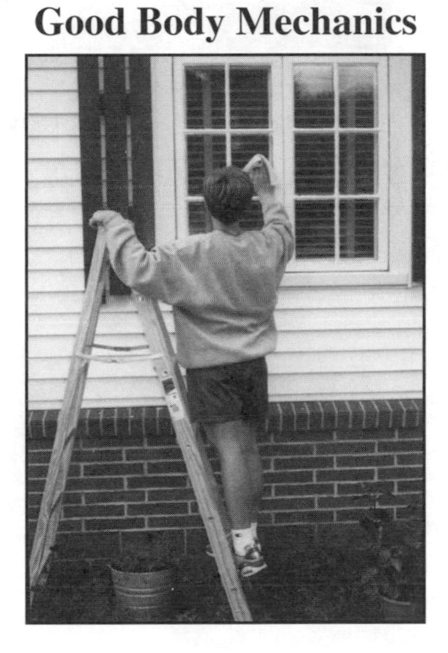

Bad Body Mechanics

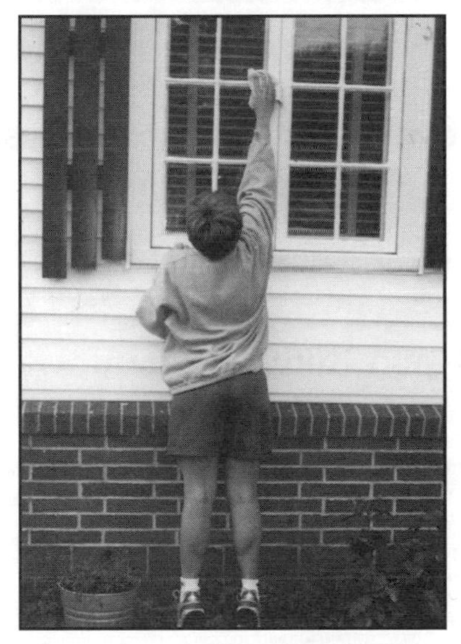

8. When carrying objects, carry two equal-in-weight objects in each hand rather than one.

   Rationale: Places less strain on your lower back muscles. It also keeps your back straight rather than tilted to one side.

Good Body Mechanics

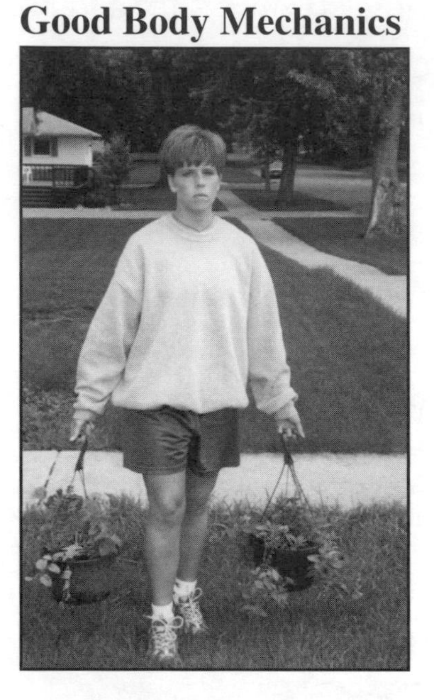

Bad Body Mechanics

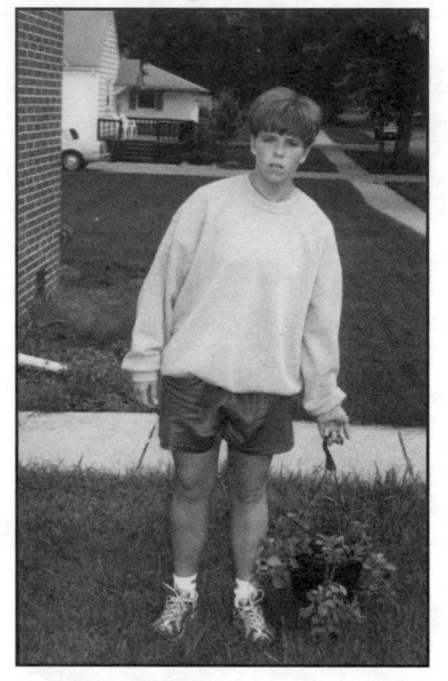

9. When digging holes to plant, use the weight of your entire body. Press down on your shovel with your leg and push down with your arms. Try and keep your back straight.

   Rationale: Places less strain on your back muscles.

Good Body Mechanics

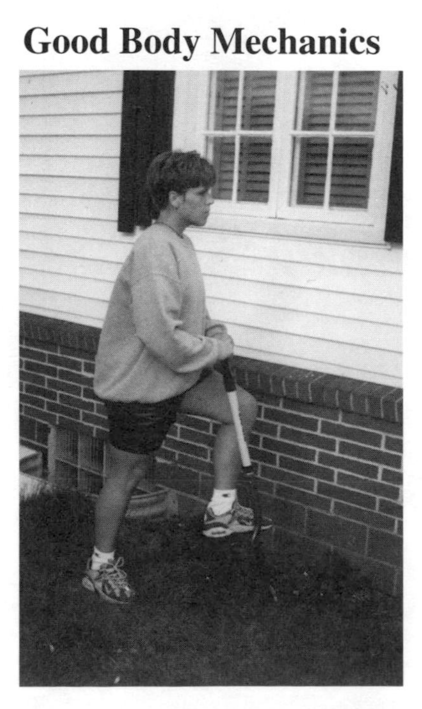

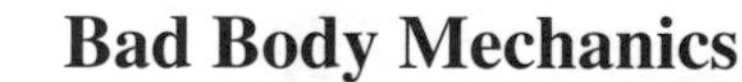

Bad Body Mechanics

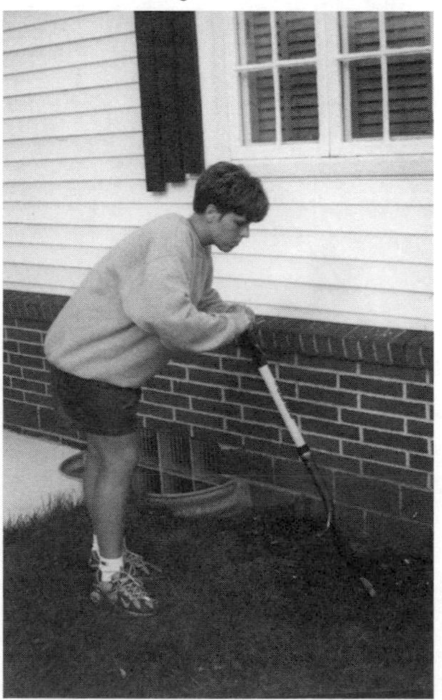

Exercises for Gardening

Standing Back Bends

Purpose: To take pressure off the back of your discs and stretch the front ligaments and muscles.

- Stand with your feet shoulder width apart.
- Place the palms of your hands on the middle of your lower back.
- Leading with your head, lean back as far as possible. Keep your knees straight during the exercise.

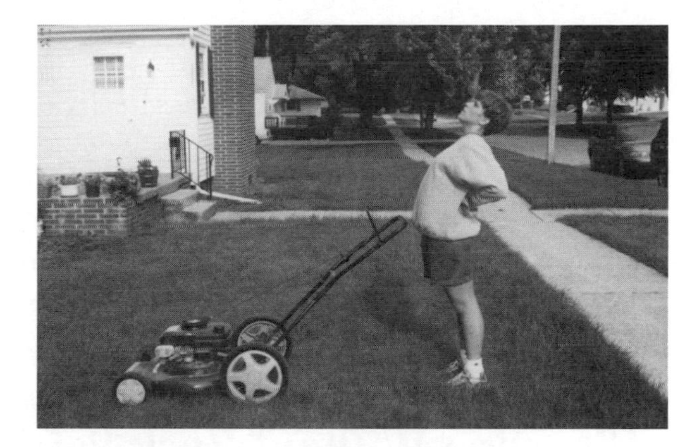

Hold for one second in the extended position and repeat 10 times. This can be repeated many times during the day to counteract the forward bending postures.

Standing Side Bend Right

Purpose: To stretch the muscles on the left side of your back.

- Place your hands on your hips.
- Bend the right side of your body towards the ground. Your right shoulder will go lower while your left shoulder should go higher.
- Do not rotate your body.

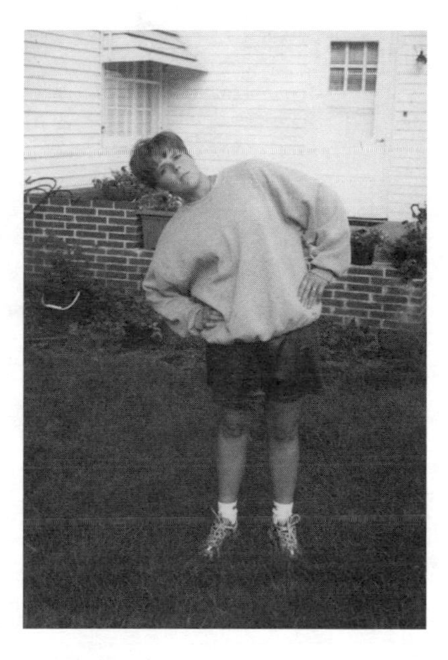

Hold for 10 seconds at the end range position. If this stretch hurts, you are probably stretching a little bit too far.

Standing Side Bend Left

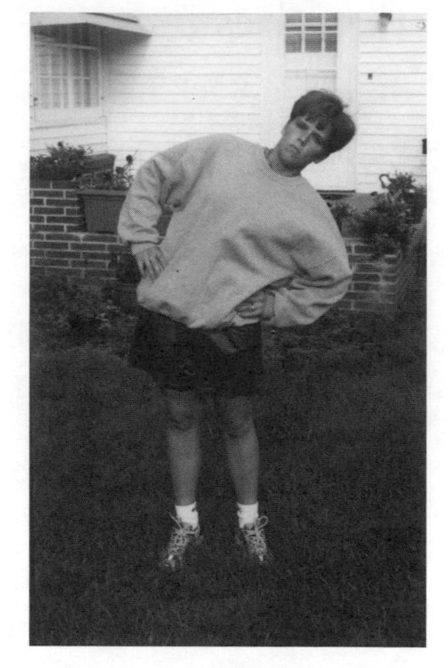

Purpose: To stretch the muscles on the right side of your back.

- Place your hands on your hips.
- Bend the left side of your body towards the ground. Your left shoulder will go lower while your right shoulder should go higher.
- Do not rotate your body.

Hold for 20 seconds at the end range position. If this stretch hurts, you are probably stretching a little bit too far.

Bicycling Without Back Pain

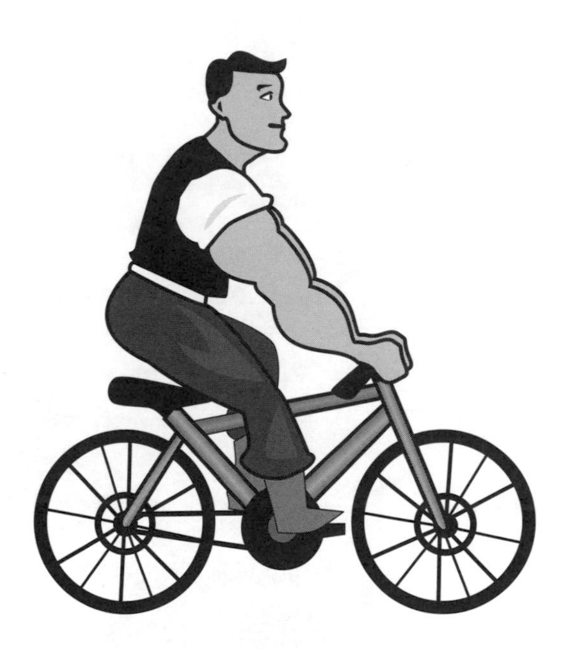

Sergio: Like many people, I love to go bicycle riding. Riding a bicycle is a relaxing and effective cardiovascular exercise, but even this low impact activity can put me at risk for a lower back injury. Here is some helpful information on how to prevent lower back pain during bicycle riding.

In order to hold on to the handlebars you have to assume the forward bending position. During bicycle riding most people bend too far forward at the waist. Maintaining this position throughout this exercise puts undo stress on your back. Here is a checklist I follow to help maintain the health of my lower back during bicycle riding.

Sergio's Bicycle Riding Checklist

1. Adjust your seat height so that you are not too high or too low.

   Rationale: Good posture during sitting is vital to preventing lower back pain. When the leg is down at its lowest position, there should be a small bend at the knee.

2. Try to maintain an upright sitting posture with a slight arch in your back.

   Rationale: Maintaining good posture will help prevent lower back discomfort. Adjust the bars to a height that will allow for an upright sitting posture.

3. Adjust your handlebars so that they are not too low.

   Rationale: Handlebars that are too low promote excessive forward bending at the waist.

Good Posture

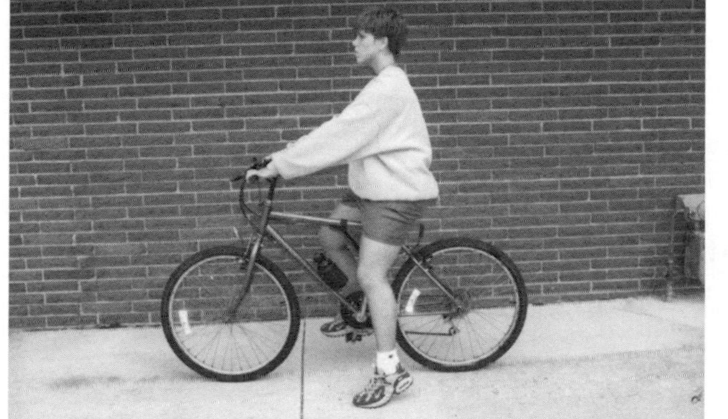

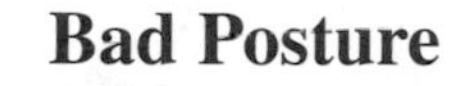

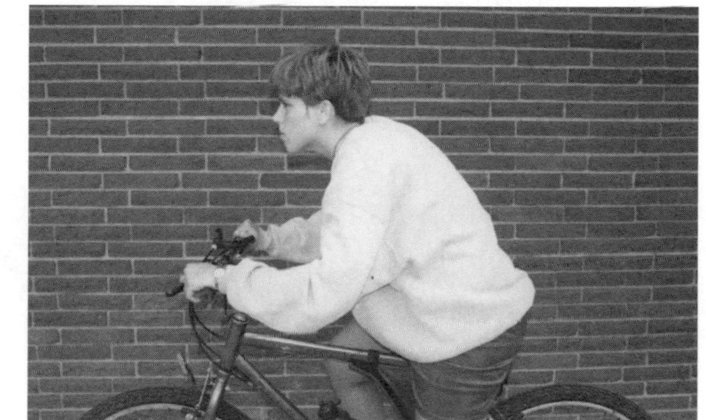

4. Get off the bike every half hour and perform one standing backbend.

   Rationale: Doing so reverses the stress placed on your lower back muscles and discs from sitting for long periods of time.

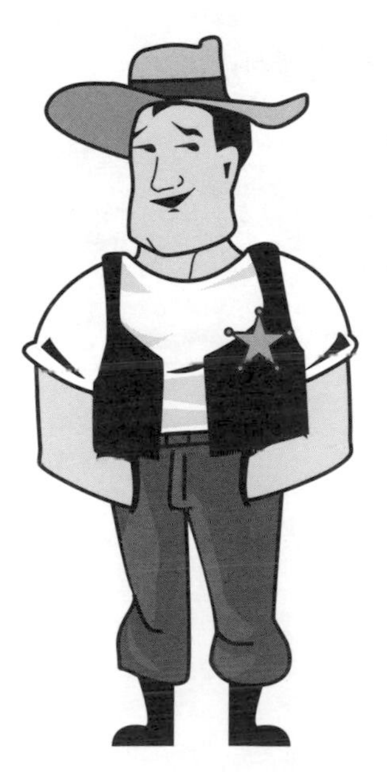

Sergio's Tip: A properly fitting seat cushion takes pressure off your tailbone.

Exercises for Bicycling

Standing Back Bends

Purpose: To take pressure off the back of your discs and stretch the front ligaments and muscles.

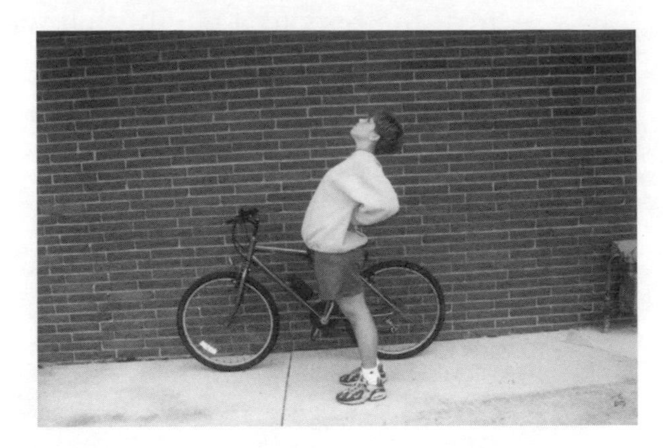

- Stand with your feet shoulders width apart.
- Place the palms of your hands on the middle of your lower back.
- Leading with your head, lean back as far as possible. Keep your knees straight during this exercise.

Hold for one second and repeat 10 times. This can be repeated many times during the day to counteract the forward bending postures.

Piriformis Stretch

Purpose: To stretch the piriformis muscle (small muscle in the middle of the buttocks), which will take pressure off the sciatic nerve.

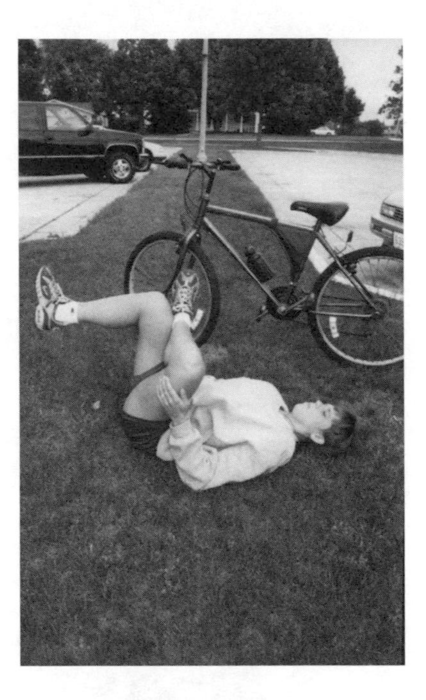

- Lie on your back with your knees bent and feet flat on the floor.
- Cross your left leg over your right just above your knee.
- Clasp your left hand behind your left knee and your right hand behind your right knee. Bring your legs toward your chest. Your legs should move together, never breaking contact with one another.
- Switch legs.

Hold for 20 seconds and repeat on the right side. You should feel a stretching sensation in the buttocks.

Standing Quadriceps Stretch

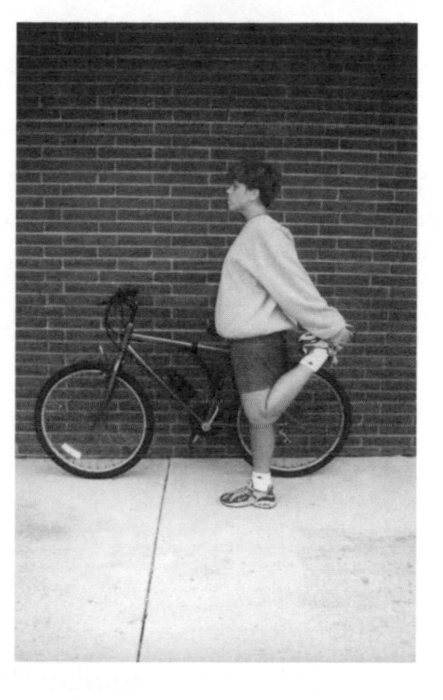

Purpose: To stretch the quadricep muscles located in the front of the thigh.

- Place your right hand on the bicycle for support and grab right above your left ankle with your left hand.
- With your left hand, help bend your knee to your buttock.

Hold for at least 20 seconds and repeat on the right side.

Standing Hamstring Stretch

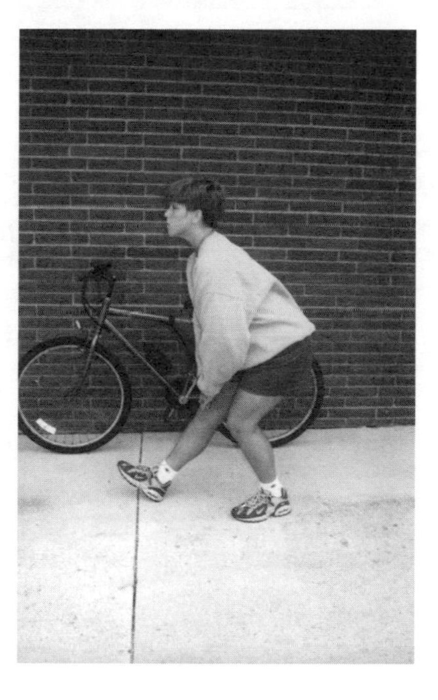

Purpose: To stretch the hamstring muscles located in the back of the thigh.

- Place your right leg straight out in front of you and slightly bend your left knee for support.
- Bend forward at the waist and slide your hands down the front of your leg. Point your toe upward.
- Bend as far forward as you can while maintaining your back straight.

Hold for at least 20 seconds and repeat on the left side.

Cooking Without Back Pain

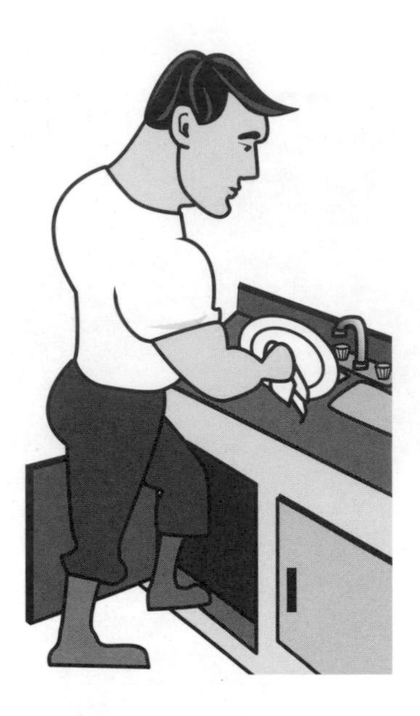

Sergio: I love to cook. I often spend Sunday afternoons in the kitchen cooking for my family and friends. Cooking relaxes me, but after a full day in the kitchen, I find myself with some stiffness in my back. Here is some helpful information on how to prevent lower back pain during cooking.

When you go to the store to buy groceries you generally have a lot of heavy bags to carry in and out of your car. Lifting heavy groceries in and out of cars puts you in an awkward physical position. When you start to cook you have to bend and reach for your pots, pans and condiments. In addition, you stand for extended periods of time. All of these activities can place undo stress on your lower back. Here is a checklist I follow to help maintain the health of my lower back while cooking.

Sergio's Cooking Checklist

1. Bend your knees, keeping a wide base of support, when moving groceries into and out of your car.

   Rationale: Good posture when lifting groceries will prevent lower back pain.

2. Wear proper kitchen attire.

   Rationale: Wearing an apron takes away the fear of spilling food on your clothes. This allows you to hold objects close your body. Holding a 10 pound pot of food away from your body places 100 pounds of stress on your spine.

3. Wear shoes that provide good support. Try to avoid wearing high heels.

   Rationale: Wearing the proper shoes takes pressure off your lower back muscles when standing for long periods.

4. If a work surface is too low, try to raise the surface.

   Rationale: This helps prevent excess forward bending of the waist and trunk.

5. Place cookbook on a bookstand that is at eye level.

   Rationale: This helps you to use good posture by keeping your head straight when reading recipes.

6. Place bookstand at a reasonable reading distance.

   Rationale: This prevents forward head posture (extending head forward) when reading your cookbook. This posture can potentially cause neck and arm pain.

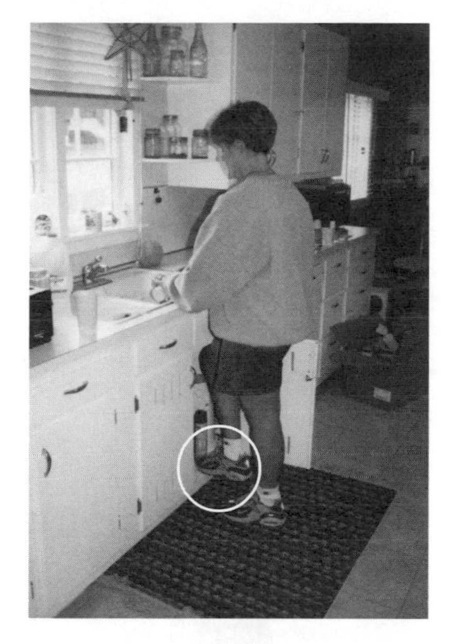

7. Place a rug under your sink to prevent wet spots.

   Rationale: This decreases the risk of slipping and falling.

8. Alternate feet on cupboard or stool when standing for long periods of time.

   Rationale: This alters the stress placed on the postural muscles of your back, preventing fatigue.

9. Alternate standing and sitting on a bar stool when cooking in a stationery position for long periods.

   Rationale: Alternating work positions shifts the stresses placed on your body, thereby reducing the likelihood of muscle fatigue.

10. Always try to sit or stand up taller than normal.

    Rationale: Doing so helps prevent a slouched posture.

11. Perform one minute of exercise every hour.

    Rationale: Periodic exercise breaks help rejuvenate your muscles and prevent muscle aches and fatigue.

Chapter 10

Causes of Lower Back Injuries: How you Hurt your Back

Microtrauma Injury

Muskull began having recurring back pain and asked Sergio for help.

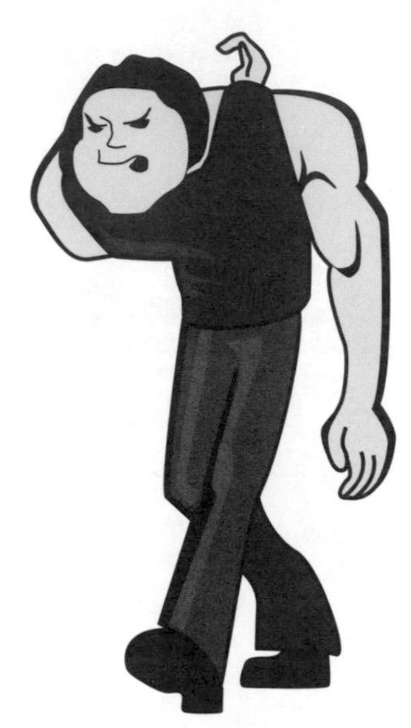

Muskull: Sergio, I am always re-injuring my lower back and I am tired of being in pain. I don't know why I hurt my back so often. What can I do to feel better?

Sergio: You may be suffering from microtrauma injuries. My best friend from college who is a well-known practitioner and educator of back treatments, provided the simplest illustration of microtrauma to me. If you take your index finger and pull it back as far as it will go, initially all you will feel is a mild stretch. If you hold that position for several minutes, eventually your finger will hurt and your natural tendency will be to let go. When you let go of your finger, the pain goes away. If you did not let go of your finger, you will start to tear some of the structures. The same can be said of some back pain episodes. For example, you may develop a backache from sitting in your car for an extended period of time. If you don't change positions, the pain will intensify and persist. If you stand when you first feel the discomfort, the pain will disappear. If you don't change your position, you may cause further damage to your spine.

Muskull: I bent over to pick up a light object and all of the sudden my back hurt.

Sergio: That is not as strange or uncommon as you may think. In fact, it happens all the time. A sudden back injury is an accumulation of many microscopic injuries that lead to one big episode of pain. Back pain is usually caused by gradual stresses on your back that accumulate over a period of time. Think of your back as a water balloon ready to burst. You can sit on the balloon, press on it with your hand, throw it at someone and the balloon might not break. If you keep abusing the balloon, eventually it will break open and the water will escape. Your back is the same way. It can take a lot of abuse. The last action you performed when injuring your back was the one your body could not handle. You cannot look inside your body to check for small microscopic injuries. Because you can still function, you don't pay attention to the little nags, aches and discomforts that accompany your everyday life. But the microtraumas continue to accumulate. You will not know the stresses placed on your back until one day you feel that disabling pain.

When you are performing an activity, whether it involves remaining in one position or moving about, if you notice any discomfort in your back then microtrauma is probably occurring. It should be a red flag to change your poor posture or body mechanics to minimize the potentially cumulative stresses to your back.

Disco: Muskull, let me give you a lesson on how I hurt my back and what I did to get better.

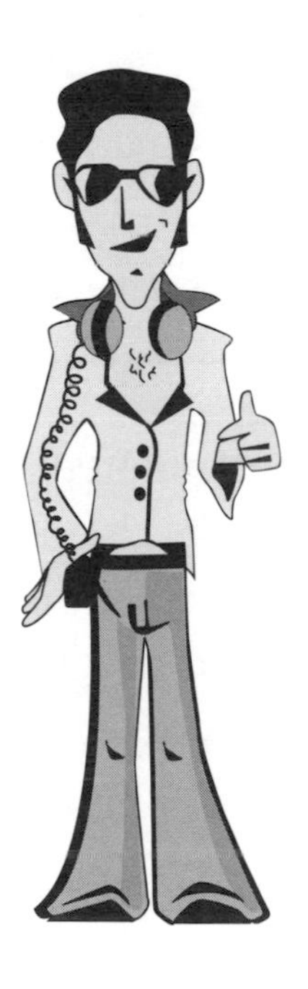

Disco's Back Lesson

When I was born, I had perfectly normal discs. As I grew up, my healthy and normal discs acted as shock absorbers for my spine. When I started school, my parents bought me a computer. I loved all the games I could play on the computer and would sit for hours at a time playing these games. Eventually, I grew up and became quite smart. However, I did not realize that the sitting I had done in school and at home in front of my computer placed my spine in an unhealthy bent forward position. This caused the fluid inside my discs to shift backward. I was young and strong and for a while could easily compensate for the damage I was causing my back. I did not realize that a bulging or herniated disc does not happen overnight and that my behavior as a youngster made me prone to a herniated disc.

During my high school years, I still had no back pain. I decided to get a construction job after school. This job was very physical and involved a lot of lifting and bending forward at the waist. I was feeling stronger than ever and did not understand the importance of good body mechanics. Each time I lifted improperly, I was pushing the disc fluid backward, thus causing more stress on the back wall of my discs.

When I graduated college, I got a job working for Sergio at his computer store. I was great at my job and was making a healthy living until one day my life changed drastically. While on the job, I bent down to pick up a computer and it finally happened! I felt a shooting pain from my back to my right foot. The fluid from one of my discs was now pressing on a nerve.

That morning, I went to see a physician, who referred me to a physical therapist. My physical therapist taught me the proper exercises I should do at work and at home in order to reverse the stress placed on my disc. He also taught me about proper posture. He demonstrated how to lift properly and how to design my workstation to minimize the stresses placed on my body. My pain diminished gradually. I was always smart and hard working, but now, most importantly,

I am **ERGONOMICALLY FIT.**

Macrotrauma Injuries

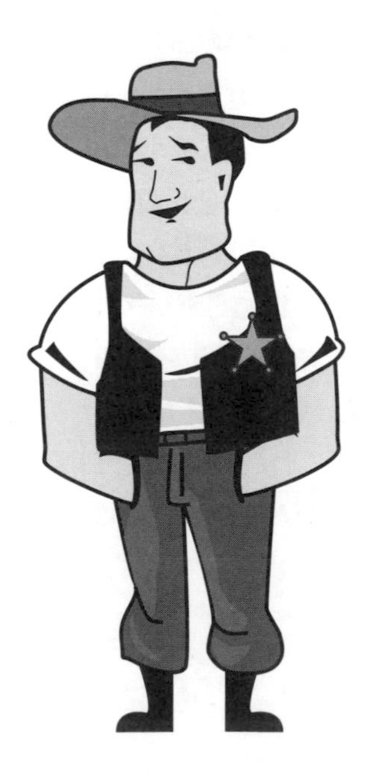

Sergio: Unlike microtrauma injuries that are accumulated stresses to your back, macrotrauma injuries happen with one single forceful event. This type of injury is easy to spot. It is usually due to a traumatic injury, such as a fall or a direct hit by an object. These “accidents” tend to leave a mark to detect where the injury took place, such as a visible cut or a broken bone. The injured area can easily be seen and identified. If the damage is not too severe, it can be fixed.

Macrotraumas can also cause pain from discs, muscle injuries or bone damage but they are closely related to a single incident and usually without prior pain. Macrotrauma injuries are caused by accidents and are usually less preventable. Whether the injury is from microtrauma or macrotrauma, the first line of treatment for pain is the same.

Muskull: What should I do if I hurt my back again?

Sergio: This is what you need to do when you first get hurt.

The best way to take care of the initial onset of pain is to remember the acronym RICE: **R**est, **I**ce, **C**ompression & **E**levation. In general, this is the most immediate, appropriate treatment when a body part such as an arm or leg is injured. The goal is to decrease inflammation and pain. When treating a back injury, a modified RICE treatment is applied: **R**est, **I**ce, **C**ompression and **E**arly Return. You can apply this early treatment principle to an injured back while you are on the phone arranging a doctor's appointment.

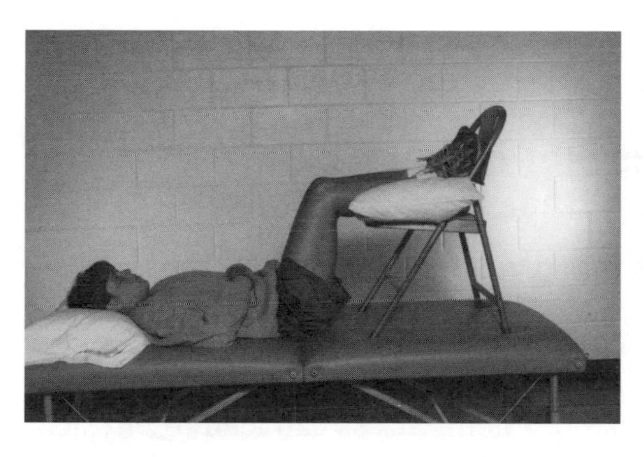

Rest: Immobilize the back. Lie in a 90/90 position (see picture below) and place an ice pack beneath the injured area of the back. This relaxes the back muscles and allows for proper healing.

Ice: Apply ice to the back for the first 24 to 48 hours. Apply the ice for 10 to 15 minutes at a time and wait at least 30 minutes before reapplying the next ice pack. Ice decreases the internal and external swelling caused by an injury.

Compression: Compression refers to the pressure you place on an injury. For back injuries, lie on your back with an ice pack beneath you and adjust your body weight so that it applies the compression needed.

Early Return: Early return to "normal" activities is important. Activities should be tolerable and not aggravating to the original injured area. Do not try to jump back into your normal routine all at once. If your back starts to hurt right away when you do return to your normal routine, you are probably overdoing it. It is important to jump back on the horse when you fall off but make sure your body is ready.

Muskull: If my pain does not disappear, when should I contact a physician?

Sergio: Here are urgent reasons to contact a physician immediately.

- If you feel a loss of muscle function, any numbness, loss of sensation or tingling in a body part.
- If you are having difficulty controlling your bowel or bladder.
- If your pain doesn't improve within 24 to 48 hours.
- If you experience pain or nausea only at night.

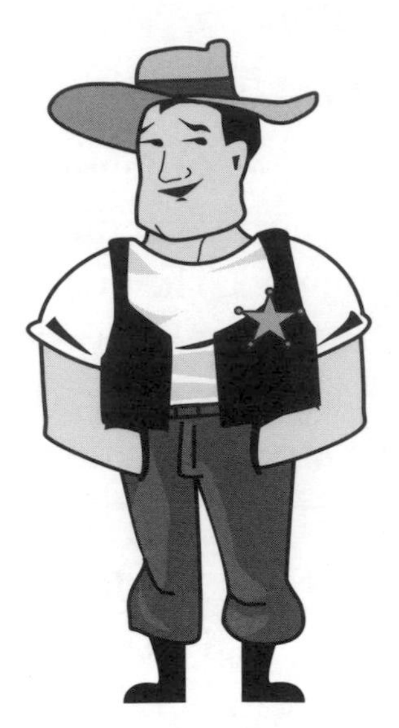

Sergio's Tip: The above are common problems seen in physical therapy and rehabilitation. If you are unsure about the origin of your back pain, consult a physician immediately.

Muskull: While we are on the subject of back pain, what else could contribute to my back hurting?

Sergio: Here are some other real risk factors for lower back pain.

Stress

Believe it or not, stress is not just an emotional problem. Stress can lead to physical injuries as well. When the body fatigues and feels stressed, the muscles tense and have to work harder and fatigue easier. This increases the likelihood for a muscle strain when performing a physical activity. This is why most athletic injuries occur during the later part of the game. Also, skiers often injure themselves in the afternoon after trying to squeeze in one last ski run. Even a rubber band will break if stretched too far. Think of yourselves as athletes at work.

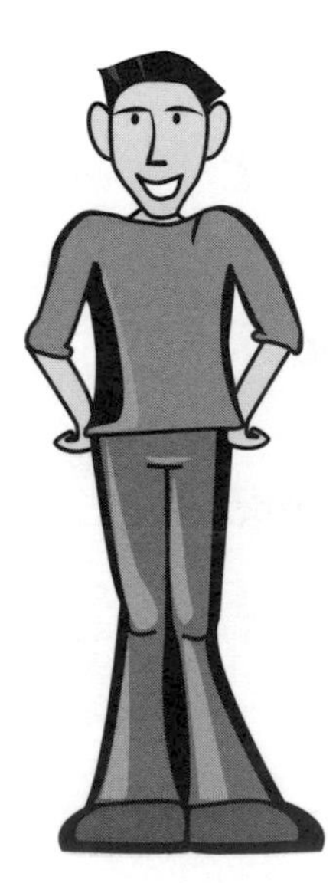

Nervie: I used to be stressed out, but now I am pain free.

Sleeping

Muskull: What is the least stressful physical position for me to sleep in?

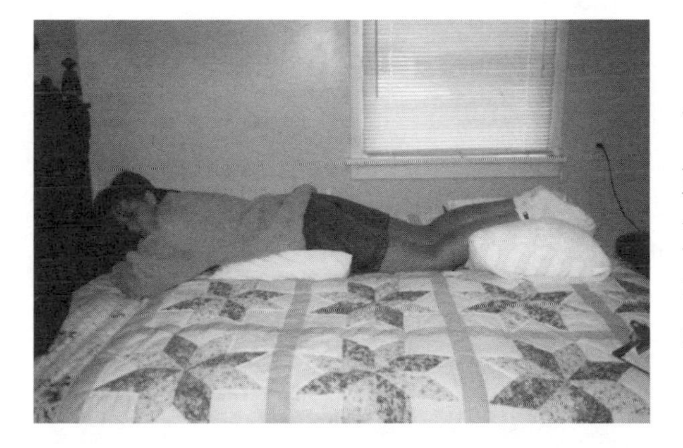

When sleeping on your stomach, place a pillow under your stomach and feet.

Note: It is adviseable for people who experience neck pain, not to sleep on their stomach.

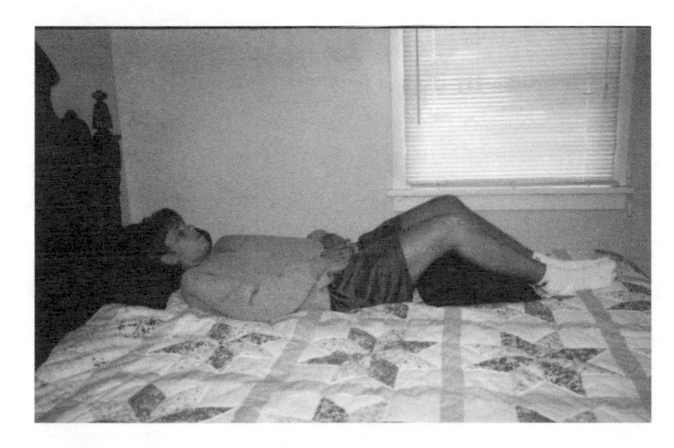

When sleeping on your back, keep your knees bent with a pillow beneath your knees.

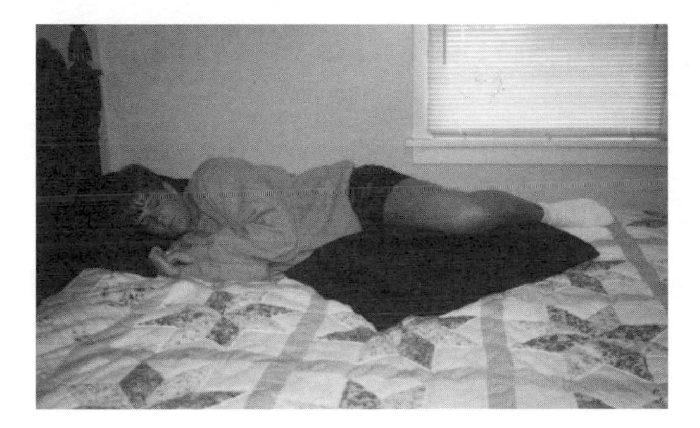

When sleeping on your side, place a pillow between your legs. The pillow helps keep the spine in neutral and the muscles most relaxed.

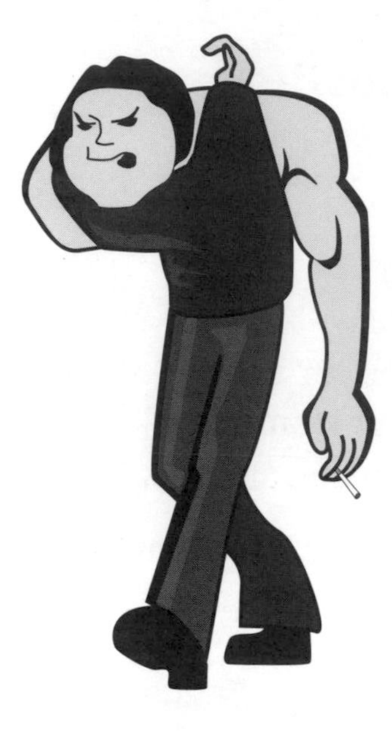

Smoking

Muskull: Does smoking have anything to do with my back pain?

Sergio: Your blood supply is your fuel. If you put poisonous carbon monoxide from smoking in your fuel supply, you will not run as well. Cigarettes also cause hardening of the arteries, which reduces the amount of blood that is transported to your muscles. Poor circulation makes the heart work more strenuously and reduces the amount of fuel your muscles receive. As a result, the muscles fatigue easier and don't heal as well from micro and macrotrauma injuries.

Muskull: Is eating right important to maintain a healthy back?

Sergio: Diet and nutrition not only affect how you look but also keep your back healthy. To help maintain an optimal blood supply, both for fuel and for waste elimination, you must have an adequate intake of vitamins and minerals. If you maintain a healthy diet, your body will work much more efficiently, than if you are on a diet loaded with junk food.

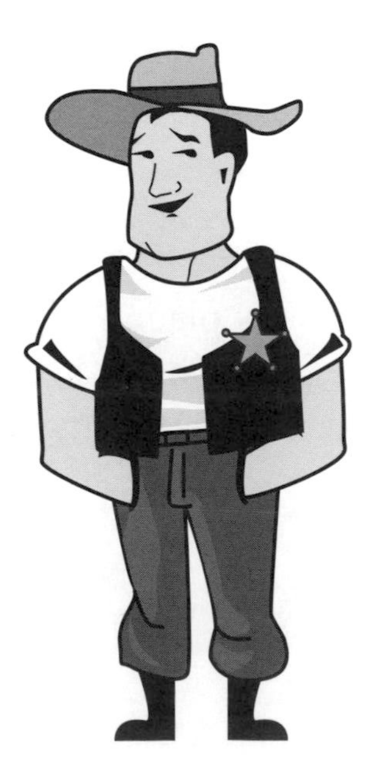

Sergio's Tip: If you want to eat healthier, buy healthier food. Buy fruits and vegetables rather than cookies and cake. Make it a rule not to shop for junk food. There is a reason they call it junk food. It's junk.

The Effects Back Pain Has on Your Life

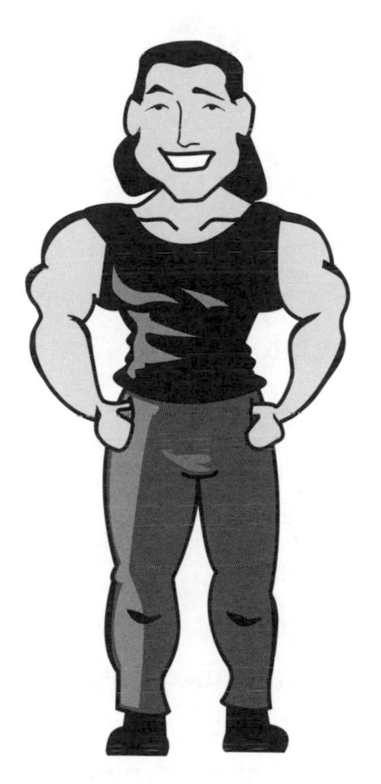

Muskull: Look at what back pain has done to me.

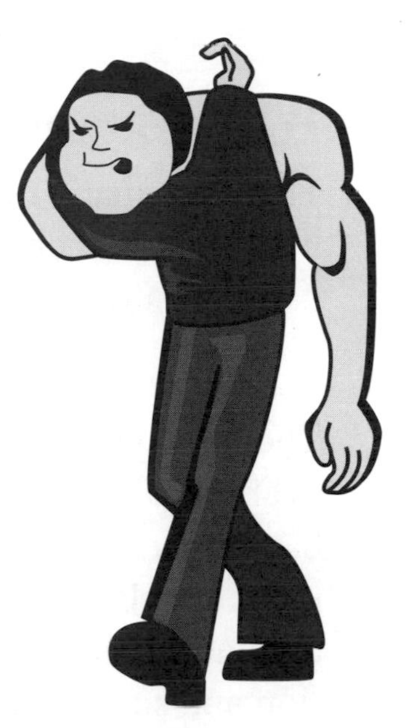

Sergio: Back pain can physically and emotionally ruin people's lives. Most people who have to leave their job because of back pain generally don't return if they are out of work for more than one year. Studies have shown approximately 90% of all people out of work for this amount of time never return. This places a heavy financial burden on the family. This can also lead to feelings of worthlessness and depression.

Back pain can also decrease one's sex drive. A person with back pain can take certain precautions during sex to avoid additional pain, however, back pain can still limit one's ability to perform sexually.

Back sufferers can also lose interest in their favorite hobbies. Those afflicted start to believe they can no longer do the things they once did. Back pain can ruin your life if you let it. A decision needs to be made. Back pain is only as debilitating as you make it. There are many avenues you can take to decrease your back pain and eventually become pain-free. Many options have been outlined in this book. The bottom line: It is up to you to control your own level of pain and discomfort.

Chapter 11

Mark and Perry's Professional Advice on Treatment for Lower Back Pain

What types of treatments are available to people with back pain?

There are many reasons for back pain. The most common have been outlined in this book. These include disc, nerve and muscle injuries. Many people may have a combination of these, as the structures of the spine are so closely interrelated.

There are various kinds of treatment for back pain and no one treatment is perfect for everyone. The most important self care treatments for back pain and prevention of back injuries have been outlined in this book. Many different kinds of formal treatment are also available including Physical Therapy, Chiropractic, Doctor of Osteopathy and Medical Doctors which include exercise, modalities, medications, manipulation and surgery. Surgery is indicated with certain conditions. Otherwise, surgery should be thought of as a last resort once a trial of proper conservative treatment has occurred.

Surgery

Surgery alone will not heal your back. Surgery should always be the last resort and should be done only after conservative treatments fail. After any surgery, the body accumulates scar tissue. Scar tissue is good because it helps the healing process by replacing older damaged tissue with new tissue. However, if you lie on your back and do nothing after surgery, this scar tissue will accumulate and grow in an abnormal formation. This accumulation of scar tissue can impinge upon a nearby nerve and cause pain. A gradual and progressive strengthening and stretching program should be initiated shortly after surgery. Knowing the "do's and don'ts" of back pain is vital to a patient's recovery. In addition, a good physical therapy program will facilitate recovery and healing.

When is surgery my last or best resort?

The best source to help you decide whether you need surgery is an orthopedist or neurological surgeon who specializes in spinal problems. Your medical doctor is a good source of other treatment choices that are available.

Certain conditions that always require surgery. They include:

1. Inability to control your bowel or bladder.

2. Weakening of the legs from one day to the next.
3. If your pain is so severe that it interferes with your everyday activities of work, walking, showering, dressing and so on.

Treating back injuries without surgery:

Physical Therapy (PT)

A physical therapist is a practitioner that commonly treats people with back pain. Generally a PT will obtain a functional history and ask you questions about your work and home activities and how these relate to your pain. Your function, strength and sensation will then objectively be assessed. Based on this information a PT will design a program that will likely include a combination of exercise and modalities such as manipulation, heat, ice, massage and electrical stimulation to relieve pain and help heal tissues. An optimal PT program is one that encourages the patient to be proactive. They work closely with doctors to establish and carry through a plan of care.

Chiropractic Doctors (DC)

These doctors are well trained in manipulation of the spine. Like physical therapists, they also use heat, ice, and stimulators to relieve pain. They are qualified and authorized to take x-rays and refer to other diagnostic tests.

Medical Doctors (MD)

Medical doctors are the same as DOs except that most are not trained in manipulations. In fact, the only major difference between DOs and MDs is that DOs gets manipulation training early in their careers. Both DOs and MDs will specialize in fields such as orthopedics, neurology, surgery, family medicine, physiatry and others.

Doctors of Osteopathy (DO)

These doctors are physicians who are trained in hands-on manipulation of the body and are licensed to take x-rays, MRIs and other tests that are used to diagnose back conditions. They can also administer medication and pain injections for relief.

Why is exercise important?

Exercise is important for preventing the occurrence or recurrence of lower back pain. A well-rounded exercise program consisting of a variety of stretching and strengthening exercises will keep your back healthy and strong. Often people wait until an injury occurs to start an exercise program. The old saying "if it ain't broke, don't fix it" is the philosophy of many people. Exercise to prevent a back injury does not entice many people. People who exercise on a daily basis are less likely to sustain a back injury.

However, exercise performed improperly could be worse than no exercise at all. We have already described to you in detail how to perform certain exercises safely and effectively. We covered a variety of exercises that are easy to do, time efficient and fun. We don't expect you to do all of the exercises. Pick out a couple of exercises from each section and perform them at least once a day. If the routine gets boring, you could always change your exercise program. After a while, this exercise routine will become a part of your life.

Education: Become an Expert

You can go to the greatest physician, physical therapist or chiropractor and leave his or her office feeling 100 % better. However, if you go back home or return to your job with the same habits that caused your pain in the first place, you will probably return to that health care professional time and again with the same complaints. To avoid frequent visits, you need to understand what causes pain and how to take care of it. In other words, proper treatment for back pain includes education.

Back pain does not happen overnight. To avoid back pain, you must establish good habits. If you incorporate these habits into your daily activities, taking proper care of your back will become a way of life. Many of our patients complain that an activity such as tennis causes them back pain. Upon interviewing the patients, we found that the back pain started two hours after they played the game. For those two hours, they sat in a lounge chair, hunched and flexed, and didn't move because they were too tired. What they didn't realize was that tennis wasn't the activity that did them in. Rather, it was the sitting posture after the activity that caused them the pain.

Modalities

The following modalities are used to speed up the healing process:

Heat: Used to increase blood flow to an injured area. This can be in the form of a warm bath, a hydrocollater pack, an electric heating pad, ultrasound, etc. These are generally used when the injury is more than two days old.

Ice: Generally used to decrease inflammation and pain at an injured area for the first 24 to 48 hours after the onset of an injury.

Ultrasound: A deep penetrating heat used specifically to flush out irritating waste products and break up accumulated scar tissue. Also promotes healing at the cellular level.

Electrical Stimulation: Used for pain relief by nerve or muscle innervation and strengthening of injured muscle. Also used to decrease edema and promote cellular healing.

Hydrotherapy: Therapy in water. Can be in the form of a swimming pool or a whirlpool. It helps loosen up the superficial muscles and allows for activities in a near weightless environment. Can also be used for strengthening, stretching and cardiovascular exercises.

Manipulation and Massage

Manipulation is used by chiropractors, physical therapists and osteopathic physicians to help readjust a malaligned spine or structure. It is used to assist in an exercise program and to regain lost joint motion. Massage is used to increase blood flow to an injured area.

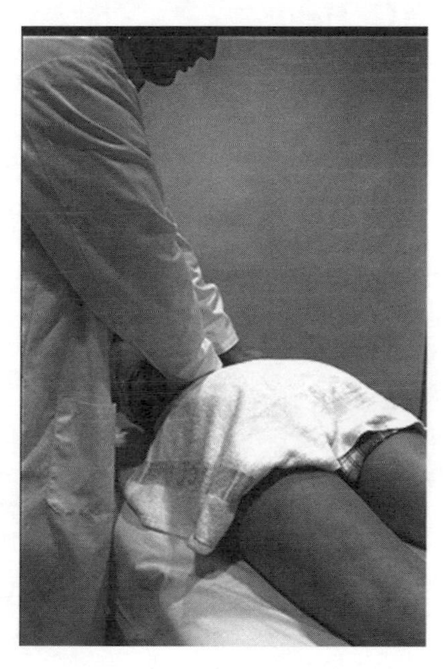

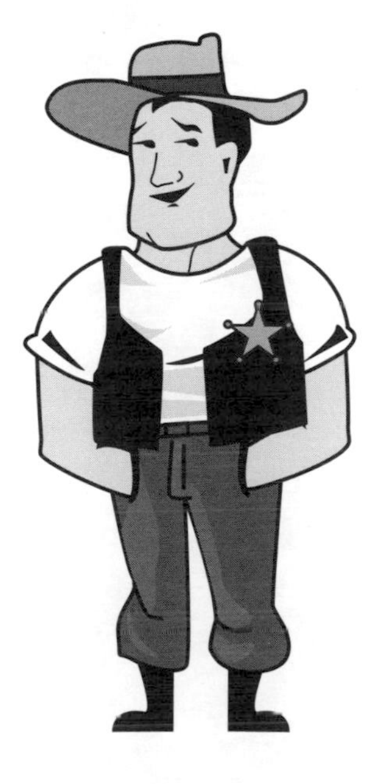

Sergio's Tip: Listen to Perry and Mark's advice. They taught me everything I know.

Chapter 12

Quiz

1. The most important patient treatment for prevention of lower back pain is:

A. Medications

B. Manipulations

C. Heat

D. Patient education

2. When you are bending forward, the fluid inside your discs moves:

A. Forward

B. Backward

C. To the left

D. To the right

3. When you are bending backward, the fluid inside your discs moves:

A. Forward

B. Backward

C. To the left

D. To the right

4. When disc fluid escapes, your disc is now:

A. Slipped

B. Bulging

C. Herniated

5. The most restful position for the lower back is:

A. 90-90 position

B. Sitting slouched

C. Standing

6. Immediately after injuring yourself, you should:

A. Apply heat

B. Apply icc

C. Neither

7. Small injuries to your back applied over a period of time is called:

A. Macrotrauma injuries

B. Microtrauma Injuries

8. When you are in slumped sitting, the fluid inside your discs moves:

A. To the left

B. To the right

C. Forward

D. Backward

9. The sciatic nerve runs from:

A. Your neck to your arm

B. Your neck to your back

C. Your lower back down to your toes

10. Ergonomics refers to:

A. The way you set up your work environment

B. The postural stresses you place on your body

C. A group of back exercises

Answer Key

1. D
2. B
3. A
4. C
5. A
6. B
7. B
8. C
9. C
10. A

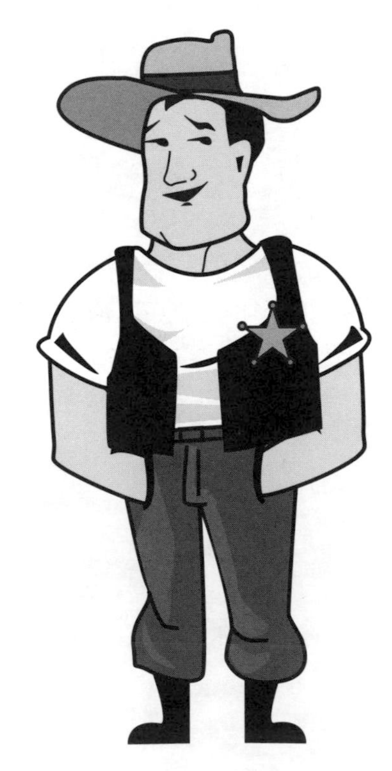

All of the answers are found in this book.

CONCLUSION

Our patients often ask us after they have finished their physical therapy program, "How am I going to maintain the health of my back now that I am done with physical therapy?" The goal of any good treatment program is delegating the responsibility of patient care to the patient. Patient education should be the first line of treatment for lower back pain. If you understand the causes of lower back pain, you will know how to take care of and treat your own back.

Unfortunately, most people do not take the time necessary to take care of their back. This is the reason that 8 out of 10 people at some time in their life will experience lower back pain. Many people wait until they are in pain to take care of themselves and then seek the quickest way to eliminate this pain. This leads to a reliance on the medical community for passive back care. As time goes on, their pain gets worse and their recovery time takes longer.

Hopefully, you have fully read and understood this book and you now know how to take care of your own back. You are empowered to preserve the life of your back. Our goal as physical therapy practitioners is to get you feeling better and to teach you how to stay healthy and fit. With our advice, your need for any future health care intervention will hopefully diminish.

You need to organize a list of all the activities causing you lower back pain. Write down the necessary changes that you need to make in order to eliminate your lower back pain. What behavioral changes are needed to decrease the likelihood of recurring lower back pain? How are you going to improve your daily posture? What exercises are you going to incorporate into your day? How are you going to change your working environment to minimize the stresses placed on your lower back? How are you going to take care of acute lower back pain so that it does not worsen? If you can answer these questions, you are well on your way to a healthier, pain-free back.

Glossary

Backward bending - This movement applies pressure on the back of the disc, pushing the fluid to the front. The fluid, being pushed forward, can cause the disc to lose its normal shape. When the disc changes shape it can press on a nerve.

Blood supply - After a long, hard day at work, irritating waste products accumulate in the muscles. This leads to muscle soreness. Ideally, your blood supply flushes out these irritating waste products, bringing the necessary vitamins and minerals to help repair and refuel the muscles. A problem arises when the muscles do not receive a great enough blood supply to help flush out the irritating waste products from the muscle.

Bulging disc - A bulging disc is when the fluid is pushed towards one side of the disc wall. The disc wall is still intact and the fluid does not escape outside of the disc.

Chiropractic Doctors (DC) - These doctors are well trained in manipulation of the spine. They also use heat, ice, and stimulators to relieve pain. They are also qualified and authorized to take x-rays and order diagnostic studies of your back to see if there are any broken bones or unusual curves of the bones.

Compression - Compression refers to the pressure you place on an injury. For back injuries, lie on your back with an ice pack beneath you and adjust your body weight so that it applies the compression needed.

Creep - Creep is when the ligaments of the back are stretched too much. If you stretch a ligament for any period of time, it lengthens and eventually develops small tears. Over time, these ligaments become weak and don't support your sitting position too well.

Doctors of Osteopathy (DO) - These are medical doctors who are trained in manipulation of the bodies musculoskeletal structures. They are also licensed to take x-rays; MRIs and other tests that are used to diagnose back conditions. They can also administer medication and pain injections for relief.

Early return - Early return to "normal" activities is important. Activities should be tolerable and not aggravating to the original injured area. Do not try jump back into your normal routine all at once. If your back starts to hurt right away when you do return to your normal routine, you are probably over doing it.

Electrical Stimulation - Can be used for pain relief by nerve or muscle innervation and strengthening of injured muscle. Also used to decrease edema and promote cellular healing.

Ergonomics - Ergonomics refers to the way you set up and interact with your work environment. If your work environment is set up ergonomically it will put less stress on the worker to perform the job.

Extension exercises - Backward bending of our spine. This movement applies pressure on the back of the disc, pushing the fluid to the front.

Flat back - When the lower back curve is decreased, you have a "flat back".

Flexion exercises - Forward bending of our spine. This movement applies pressure on the front of the disc, pushing the fluid to the back.

Forward bending - Forward bending applies pressure on the front of the disc. This pressure pushes the fluid to the back of the disc. The fluid, being pushed backward, can cause the disc to lose its normal shape. When the disc changes shape it can press on a nerve.

Herniated disc - A herniated disc is one step worse than a bulge. This is when the fluid escapes and breaks through the disc wall.

Hydrotherapy - Therapy in water. Can be in the form of a swimming pool or a whirlpool. It helps loosen up the (superficial muscles) and allows for activities in a near weightless environment. Can also be used for strengthening exercises.

Ice - It is generally used to decrease inflammation and pain to an injured area for the first 24 to 48 hours of the onset of an injury.

Lumbar lordosis - The curve in your lower back is called your lumbar lordosis.

Macrotrauma injury - Macrotrauma injuries happen with one single forceful event. This type of injury is easy to spot. It is usually due to a traumatic injury, such as a fall or a direct hit by an object. These "accidents" tend to leave a mark to detect where the injury took place, such as a visible cut or a broken bone. The injured area can easily be seen and identified. If the damage is not too severe, it can be fixed.

Medical Doctors (MD) - These medical doctors are the same as the DO except that most are not trained in manipulations. In fact, the only major difference between DO's (Doctors of Osteopathy) and MD's (Medical Doctors) is that the DO gets manipulation training early in their careers. Both DO's and MD's go will specialize in fields such as Orthopedics, Neurology, Surgery, Family Medicine, Physiatry and others.

Microtrauma injury - A sudden back injury is an accumulation of many microscopic injuries that lead to one big episode of pain. Back pain is usually caused by gradual stresses on your back that accumulate over a period of time. The last action you performed when injuring your back was the one your body could no longer handle.

Muscle spasm - A muscle spasm is your body's way of telling you to slow down before you get seriously hurt. Generally, muscle aches prevent you from continuing a particular activity that would be harmful. This is known as "muscle guarding." A spasm is triggered when you consistently decrease the blood flow to a muscle ("decreased circulation"). This happens when you overwork your muscles and do not provide them with sufficient rest.

Muscle strain - As a muscle becomes tired, it tightens, and loses its flexibility becoming more susceptible to injury. You are more likely to strain a tight muscle than a loose muscle. A muscle that is constantly at work will continue to tighten. It will injure if it is not stretched regularly.

Nerves - Nerves are sensitive fibers that are responsible for sending information to muscles to carry out movement, interpret sensation and protect us by monitoring our systems and our surroundings.

Normal lumbar lordosis - If you have a normal curve in your spine, the small joints of your back are at a normal distance from one another. There is less likelihood for your muscles to tighten and the disc fluid is evenly distributed.

Physical Therapy - A physical therapist will measure your movement, strength and sensation. A therapist will ask you questions about your work, home activities and how and where the pain originated. Based on this, a therapist will usually recommend a treatment that will include exercises. Besides the exercises, therapists use heat, ice, manipulation, massage and stimulators to relieve pain and help tissues heal.

Referred pain - Referred pain is felt at a location other than the actual problem area. You might experience pain and numbness down your leg into your foot. Is the problem area in your foot or is it in your back? Nerves exiting your spinal cord in your lower back travel all the way down to your toes. You can have a pinched nerve in the back, yet the pain sensation may occur anywhere that the nerve travels, including the lower legs.

RICE treatment - **R**est, **I**ce, **C**ompression & **E**levation. An injured arm or leg requires rest, ice, compression and elevation to decrease inflammation and pain. You can apply this early treatment principle to an injured back while you are on the phone arranging a doctor's appointment. When treating a back injury, a modified RICE treatment is applied: **R**est, **I**ce, **C**ompression & **E**arly Return.

Sciatic - The sciatic is a group of nerves that run from your lower back down to your toes. A herniated or bulging disc, or inflamed joints in the back may press on it, causing shooting pain, tingling or numbness from the back or buttocks down the leg.

Sleeping - When sleeping on your back, keep your knees bent with a pillow beneath your knees. When sleeping on your side, place a pillow between your legs. When sleeping on your stomach, place a pillow under your stomach.

Smoking - Your blood supply is your fuel. If you put poisonous carbon monoxide in your fuel supply, you will not run as well. Cigarettes also cause hardening of the arteries, which reduces the amount of blood that is transported to your muscles. Poor circulation makes the heart work more strenuously and reduces the amount of fuel your muscles receive.

Stress - When the body fatigues and feels stressed, the muscles tense and have to work harder. This increases the likelihood for a muscle strain when you get up and perform a physical activity. This is why most athletic injuries occur during the later period of a game.

Surgery - Surgery alone will not heal your back. Surgery should always be the last resort and only after conservative treatments fail. After any surgery, the body accumulates scar tissue. Scar tissue is good because it helps the healing process by replacing older damaged tissues with new tissues. However, if you lie on your back and do nothing after surgery, this scar tissue will accumulate and grow in an abnormal formation. This accumulation of scar tissue will potentially impinge upon a nearby nerve and cause pain. A gradual and progressive strengthening and stretching program should be initiated shortly after surgery. Knowing the "do's" and "don'ts" of back pain is also vital to a patient's recovery. In addition, a good physical therapy program will facilitate recovery and healing.

Sway back - When the lower back curve is increased, you have a "sway back".

Ultrasound - A deep penetrating heat used specifically to flush out irritating waste products and break up accumulated scar tissue. Also promotes healing at the cellular level and helps break up adhesions and scarring.

Bibliography

1. Bullock, M. “Ergonomics: The Physiotherapist in the Workplace.” Churchill Livingstone, 1990.

2. Caplan, D. “Back Trouble.” Gainesville, Triad Publishing Co., 1987.

3. Frymoyer, J. “Helping Your Patients Avoid Low Back Pain.” Journal of Musculoskeletal Medicine. February, 1984.

4. Gray, H. “Anatomy of the Human Body.” Philadelphia, Lea & Febiger, 1936.

5. Hart, D. “Effects of Lumbar Posture on Lifting.” Spine. Vol. 12, No. 2.

6. Hickey, D. “Relation Between Structure of the Annulus Fibrosus and the Function and Failure of the Intervertebral Disc.” Spine. Vol. 5, No. 2. Magee, DJ. “Orthopedic Physical Assessment.” Philadelphia, W.B. Saunders, 1992.

7. McKenzie, R. “The Lumbar Spine.” New Zealand, Spinal Publications, Ltd., 1981.

8. McKenzie, R. “Treat Your Own Back.” New Zealand, Spinal Publications, Ltd., 1985.

9. White, AA III. “Your Aching Back.” Toronto, Bantam, 1983.

Index

About the Authors

Mark Amir MAPT, Dip MDT

Mr. Amir graduated Touro College in 1993 with a Masters degree in physical therapy. Mark has spent his professional career treating patients with various musculoskeletal problems. Recently, Mark has focused his skills on treating patients with spine conditions. The main goal of his treatment is to empower patients to treat themselves and avoid future recurrence of injuries. This also consists of counseling and consulting major corporations on instituting injury prevention and safety programs for their non-injured employees. Mark lectures at several hospitals and has taught at Bergen Community College in New Jersey. Mark received his diploma in Mechanical Diagnosis and Therapy from the McKenzie Institute International. This is the organization's highest recognized level of achievement in treating patients with musculoskeletal injuries. In the future, Mark would like to see physical therapists spend more of their efforts on finding functional solutions for their patients, rather than making them dependent on the therapist for care.

Perry Bonomo MAPT

Mr. Bonomo graduated Touro College in 1993 with a Masters degree in physical therapy. Perry is co-owner of two orthopedic private practices in New Milford, New Jersey and Brooklyn, NY. He is the senior ergonomics trainer for ErgAerobics Inc. Perry specializes in treating patients with repetitive stress injuries and teaches back, neck-arm and ergonomic seminars at various hospitals and corporations. Perry is certified at performing Functional Capacity Evaluations (FCEs), which are used to determine the level at which an injured worker is capable of returning to work. He also has certifications to perform Worksite Analyses and OSHA 10-hour and 30-hour safety programs. Perry co-founded ErgAerobics Inc., co-authored Why Does Working @ My Computer Hurt So Much? and produced the Ergercise video.

For other great Injury Prevention products and services available from **ErgAerobics**, contact us at www.ergaerobics.com info@ergaerobics.com or 800.689.9199

Order Form

Qty		Total
	ErgAerobics: Why does my back hurt so much? $14.95 A comprehensive guide to prevent and treat lower back pain. The book is easy to understand, educational, and entertaining.	
	ErgAerobics: Why does working @ my computer hurt so much? $14.95 A comprehensive guide to prevent and treat Computer Induced Repetitive Stress Injuries. The book is easy to understand, educational, and entertaining.	
	The ErgErcise Video $14.95 An instructional 25-minute video of 42 effective and inconspicuous ErgErcises that are easy to perform right at your workstation. The ErgErcise Video will teach you how to prepare your body for the computer revolution.	
	ErgAerobics Ergercise Poster $3.95 An 11"X17" glossy with 8 essential ErgErcises.	
	Subtotal	
	Please add applicable sales tax	
	TOTAL	

Payment Method: __Check __Visa __Master Card __American Express

Credit Card # ____________________ Exp. Date ___/___ Billing City and Zip__________________

Name__________________________ Address________________________ e-mail__________________

City______________________ State____ Zip__________ Phone#(___)____-________________